Case Studies in Neurology for the House Officer

Case Studies in Neurology for the House Officer

Adapted from
Intensive Clinical Neurology Course (ICNC)

Stephen L. Hauser, M.D.
Instructor in Neurology
Harvard Medical School
Boston, Massachusetts

Lawrence P. Levitt, M.D.
Chief, Division of Neurology
Allentown Hospital and
Lehigh Valley Hospital Center
Allentown, Pennsylvania

Howard L. Weiner, M.D.
Robert L. Kroc Associate Professor of
Neurologic Diseases
Brigham and Women's Hospital
Harvard Medical School
Boston, Massachusetts

WILLIAMS & WILKINS
Baltimore • Hong Kong • London • Sydney

Editor: John N. Gardner
Associate Editor: Carol Eckhart
Design: JoAnne Janowiak
Illustration Planning: Joseph Cummings
Production: Anne G. Seitz

Williams & Wilkins
428 East Preston Street
Baltimore, MD 21202, U.S.A.

Accurate indications, adverse reactions, and dosage schedules for drugs are provided in this book, but it is possible that they may change. The reader is urged to review the package information data of the manufacturers of the medications mentioned.

Printed in the United States of America

Library of Congress Cataloging in Publication Data

Main entry under title:
Hauser, Stephen L.
Case studies in neurology for the house officer.
Companion v. to; Neurology for the house officer/Howard L. Weiner, Lawrence P. Levitt. 3rd ed. c1983.
Includes index.
1. Nervous system—Diseases—Case studies. 2. Neurology—Case studies. I. Levitt, Lawrence P., 1940– . II. Weiner, Howard L. III. Weiner, Howard L. Neurology for the house officer. 3rd ed. IV. Title. [DNLM: 1. Neurologic Manifestations—case studies. 2. Neurology—case studies. WL 100 H3755c]
RC355.W44 1983 Suppl. 616.8′.09 85-9533
ISBN 0-683-03899-0

90 91 92 93 94 8 7 6 5 4 3 2

To the house officers whom we have had the pleasure of teaching and learning from over the years.

Foreword

It is indeed a pleasure to write the foreword for _Case Studies in Neurology for the House Officer_. This volume is, in a sense, the offspring of _Neurology for the House Officer_ and _Pediatric Neurology for the House Officer_. Stephen L. Hauser has joined Lawrence P. Levitt and Howard L. Weiner for what I am sure will be another very successful effort at teaching neurology.

Neurology has traditionally been the most poorly understood discipline taught in medical school. One reason is the inherent complexity of the nervous system. Another cause has been poor teaching of neurology, often couched in mysterious language and isolated from reality. Yet neurology has entered a new era characterized by a rapid expansion of knowledge in understanding the pathophysiologic basis of nervous system diseases and by increasingly effective treatment modalities. Every physician and surgeon must now be familiar with the major categories of neurologic disease.

Recently, there has been an increased effort to teach medicine by the case study approach. At the Harvard Medical School, we are presently engaged in a major project called The New Pathway, in which all aspects of medicine - from basic science to clinical work - will be taught to students using case studies. *Case Studies in Neurology for the House Officer* is thus timely, written by utilizing carefully selected, authentic case histories to emphasize seminal issues in neurologic medicine. The cases make the material memorable. It is almost as if one had seen the case oneself, adding, as it were, to one's own clinical experience by reading the book.

I am confident that this method, which is well suited to neurology, will be adopted by many other disciplines when the inevitable success of this book becomes evident.

Martin A. Samuels, M.D.
Harvard Medical School
Boston, Massachusetts

About the Authors

<u>Stephen L. Hauser, M.D.</u>, currently is a Visiting Scientist at the Pasteur Institute and Consultant in Neurology at the Salpetriere Hospital in Paris, France. A graduate of the Massachusetts Institute of Technology and the Harvard Medical School, Dr. Hauser then trained in internal medicine at Cornell Medical School and in neurology at the Massachusetts General Hospital. Beginning in 1986, Dr. Hauser will be Director of the Neuroimmunology Unit at the Massachusetts General Hospital and Assistant Professor of Neurology at the Harvard Medical School.

<u>Lawrence P. Levitt, M.D.</u>, is Chief of the Division of Neurology at the Allentown Hospital and the Lehigh Valley Hospital Center in Allentown, Pennsylvania, and is an Associate in Neurology at the University of Pennsylvania School of Medicine, and Clinical Associate Professor of Neurology at Temple University School of Medicine. A graduate of Queens College, he then attended Cornell Medical College as a Jonas Salk Scholar. Dr. Levitt interned and was a first-year medical resident at Bellevue Hospital and then spent two years in the Public Health Service at the Encephalitis Research Center in Tampa, Florida. He did his neurology training at the Harvard teaching hospitals of the Longwood Area Neurology Program.

<u>Howard L. Weiner, M.D.</u>, is Associate in Medicine (Neurology) at the Brigham and Women's Hospital and Robert L. Kroc Associate Professor of Neurologic Diseases at the Harvard Medical School. He attended Dartmouth College and the University of Colorado Medical School; he then interned at Chaim Sheba Hospital, Tel Hashomer, Israel, and served as a medical resident at the Beth

Israel Hospital, Boston. Dr. Weiner is Director of the Multiple Sclerosis Clinical and Research Unit and Co-Director of the Center for Neurologic Diseases at the Brigham and Women's Hospital.

With a foreword by Martin Samuels, M.D.

Martin A. Samuels is Associate Professor of Neurology at the Harvard Medical School and Chief of the Neurology Service at the Brockton-West Roxbury Veterans Administration Medical Center. As an internist and neurologist, he has been interested in the neurological aspects of general medical disease, particularly the relationship between brain and heart disease. He has been intimately involved in the teaching of neurology to medical students, residents, and postgraduate physicians, and is involved in the writing of a new case oriented curriculum for the Harvard Medical School. He is the author of numerous articles concerning the medical aspects of neurologic diseases and is the editor of The Manual of Neurologic Therapeutics.

Preface

In 1974 the first edition of Neurology for the House Officer was published. That manual, designed to guide medical students and house officers to properly recognize and treat neurologic disease, was enthusiastically received and required seven reprintings in three years. The second edition appeared in 1978, was translated into several foreign languages, and the third edition appeared in 1983.

The enthusiastic response to Neurology for the House Officer led to the Intensive Clinical Neurology Course (ICNC) designed to provide a course for non-neurologists which emphasized a problem-oriented approach to common neurologic problems. The course was first held in New York City in March, 1978. It had a case history format, from patients we had seen, followed by pertinent questions and key points or "pearls" for each neurologic subject. The emphasis was on problem solving rather than the traditional didactic approach, although we also included useful factual information.

The course proved very popular and has been repeated yearly since 1978. Several of those who attended the course asked if the course syllabus might be expanded to include a wide spectrum of clinical cases that illustrate important clinical neurologic principles. Case Studies in Neurology for the House Officer is our response to those requests. We have compiled cases from our practices which illustrate key problems and lessons in neurology. Some cases are easy to diagnose and are included to represent important clinical conditions. Other cases are diagnostic dilemmas designed to challenge the reader. All cases have questions related to the cases, "pearls," and "pitfalls". In addition, most cases have a "clue" in the form of a diagram or CT scan. Although not a textbook, upon finishing this case history book, readers will have been exposed to a majority of the categories of neurologic diseases they are likely to encounter in their clinical practices and will have been taught salient points about each case. Thus, we see this case history book as a companion to _Neurology for the House Officer_ and as a "clinical textbook" in which physicians can test their neurologic acumen on actual cases. If you can recognize and diagnose each of the cases in this book and learn the pearls and pitfalls associated with them, you will have a base of clinical neurologic skills from which to continue learning neurology as you encounter patients with neurologic illness.

Stephen L. Hauser, M.D.
Lawrence P. Levitt, M.D.
Howard L. Weiner, M.D.

Acknowledgements

This manual was reviewed by students and house officers at the Harvard teaching hospitals of the Longwood Area Neurology Program and at the Allentown Hospital and Lehigh Valley Hospital Center. We are grateful to them for their encouragement, enthusiasm, and advice, and for identifying those neurologic problems and concepts most important to them. We would like to especially thank the following members of the neurology staff and house staff for their help and for reviewing parts of the manuscript: Paul Guillard, Stewart Tepper, and John Carter. We would also like to thank Rachel Kreithen and Pam Battiglino for their assistance with the illustrations, and Pat Lamy for preparation of the manuscript.

Contents

FLUCTUATING DIPLOPIA

CASE 1: A 32-year-old woman presented with a 1-month history of diplopia. She had noted intermittent horizontal diplopia which seemed to vary during the day and was usually worse in the evening. She also reported episodes of slurred speech and occasional drooping of her left eyelid. Six years previously she had an operation for "an overactive thyroid gland" and since then has been maintained on thyroid replacement. Family history was noncontributory.

Examination included normal vital signs and general physical examination. She had bilateral ptosis, worse on the left; ptosis worsened after 20 seconds of sustained upgaze. Pupils were 3 mm, horizontal eye movements were limited to several millimeters in either direction on the left; on the right, adduction was complete but abduction was decreased 50%. Vertical eye movements were intact. Musculature of face, jaw, palate and tongue were strong, and facial sensation was normal. The remainder of motor, sensory and reflex examination was normal.

NEUROANATOMICAL CLUE:

The muscles of eye opening (levator palpebrae) and eye closure (orbicularis oculi) are innervated by cranial nuclei at different levels of the brainstem; weakness of both eye opening and closure in an alert patient suggests that the disorder is outside of the brainstem and in the peripheral nervous system (nerve, neuromuscular junction, or muscle). The absence of sensory symptoms or signs makes a neuropathy unlikely.

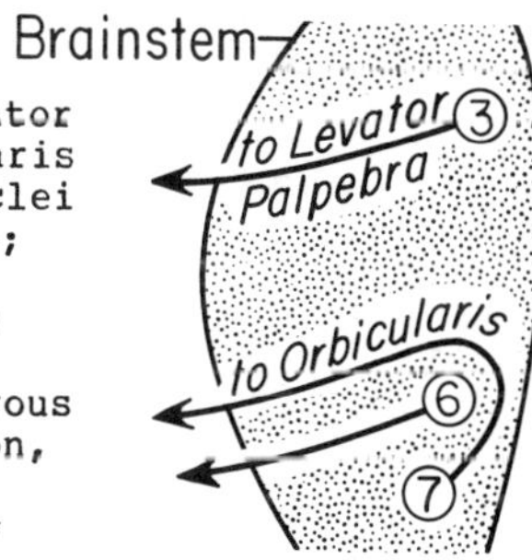

QUESTIONS:

1. What is the diagnosis? Patients with this disease are usually classified into four categories. Please name them.

2. What is the most common presenting feature of this illness?

3. What medication is used to confirm the diagnosis? What is its mechanism of action? What other laboratory tests are indicated?

4. What is the appropriate treatment for this disease?

5. What is the current theory of pathogenesis?

ANSWERS:

1. Myasthenia gravis. Group 1) ocular; 2a) mild generalized; 2b) moderate generalized; 3) acute fulminating; 4) late, severe.

2. Eye signs due to involvement of the levator palpebrae (ptosis) and extraocular muscles (diplopia) are the most common presenting features and appear at some time in over 90% of patients. Other muscle groups commonly involved include those of facial expression, chewing, swallowing, speech, neck, and proximal limbs.

3. An intravenous injection of edrophonium chloride (Tensilon), a short-acting anticholinesterase agent, will improve or reverse symptoms in most patients. Electromyography (EMG) demonstrates a characteristic pattern, consisting of a decremental response of the compound action potential to repetitive nerve stimulation at 3/second.

4. Many myasthenic patients are controlled on anticholinesterase medication alone. Thymectomy, mandatory for those patients with malignant thymoma, usually improves symptoms in patients with or without thymoma. Alternate day corticosteroids are useful and are often used in conjunction with thymectomy. Plasmapheresis has been used with initial success, but is recommended only for short-term stabilization of severe myasthenic symptoms. Immunosuppressive agents, e.g., azathioprine and cyclophosphamide, are reserved for patients refractory to other treatments.

5. Symptoms are the result of an antibody-mediated, autoimmune attack on the postsynaptic portion of the neuromuscular junction. Ninety percent of patients have circulating antibodies against one or several postsynaptic structures (acetylcholine receptor site, extrajunctional receptor, striated muscle). Antibody and complement are present at the neuromuscular junction in myasthenia. In addition, myasthenia can be transferred to animals by injecting immunoglobulin from myasthenic patients and transient "neonatal myasthenia" occurs in 12% of infants born to myasthenic mothers due to transplancental transfer of immunoglobulin.

PEARLS:

1. Malignant thymomas occur in 15% of myasthenics (more commonly in older males). Of patients without thymoma, 80% have thymic hyperplasia. All patients with myasthenia require a complete evaluation for thymoma including, if possible, a CT scan of the mediastinum.

2. Patients with myasthenia gravis have a higher incidence of other autoimmune disorders, including thyrotoxicosis, rheumatoid arthritis, systemic lupus erythematosus, and polymyositis.

3. A decremental EMG response occurs when normal muscle is stimulated at a rate of 20/second; decremental responses at slower rates of stimulation are typical for myasthenia and botulism.

4. Weakness in myasthenia fluctuates; other causes of fluctuating or recurrent muscular weakness include the periodic paralyses (hypokalemic, normokalemic, hyperkalemic varieties).

5. Young women with myasthenia gravis have an increased incidence of the histocompatibility type HLA-A8.

6. Although the presence of anti-acetylcholine receptor antibodies in serum is diagnostic of myasthenia gravis, the levels of antibody present do not correlate with the severity of disease.

PITFALLS:

1. Some patients, particularly those with ocular myasthenia, may not respond to anticholinesterase agents; a negative Tensilon test does not exclude the diagnosis of myasthenia.

2. Patients with myasthenia may worsen when given a variety of antibiotics including kanamycin, streptomycin, and tetracycline.

3. Temporary worsening of myasthenia may occur when beginning high-dose steroid therapy; if possible, low doses of alternate day steroids should be used initially with gradual increases as required.

4. The patient with worsening symptoms and increasing anticholinesterase requirements presents a special problem. Excessive anticholinesterase effect (<u>cholinergic crisis</u>) may resemble myasthenic crisis. Often all medications must be temporarily discontinued and the patient closely observed in an intensive care unit.

REFERENCES

1. Drachman DB: Myasthenia gravis. N Engl J Med 298 (Pt 1): 136-142, (Pt 2):186-193, 1978.
2. Engel AG, Lambert EH, Howard FM Jr: Immune complexes (IgG and C3) at the motor endplate in myasthenia gravis: ultrastructural and light microscopic localization and electrophysiologic correlations. Mayo Clin Proc 52:267, 1977.
3. Kelly JJ: The laboratory diagnosis of mild myasthenia gravis. Ann Neurol 12:238, 1982.
4. Kimura J: Principles and pitfalls of nerve conduction studies. Ann Neurol 16:415, 1984.
5. Seybold ME, Drachman DB: Gradually increasing doses of prednisone in myasthenia gravis; reducing the hazards of treatment. N Engl J Med 290:91, 1974.
6. Stefannson K, Dieperink ME, Richman DP, Gomez CM, Marton LS: Sharing of antigenic determinants between the nicotinic acetylcholine receptor and proteins in escherichia coli, proteus vulgaris, and klebsiella pneumoniae: possible role in the pathogenesis of myasthenia gravis. N Engl J Med 312:221, 1985.
7. Toyka KV, Drachman DB, Griffin DE, et al: Myasthenia gravis: study of humoral immune mechanisms by passive transfer to mice. N Engl J Med 296:125, 1977.
8. Tzartos SJ, Seybold ME, Lindstrom JM: Specificities of antibodies to acetylcholine receptors from myasthenia gravis patients measured with monoclonal antibodies. Proc Natl Acad Sci USA 79:188, 1982.

NUMBNESS AND ATAXIA

CASE 2: A 65-year-old Contessa was referred because of numbness. Six years earlier she noted a "strange" feeling in her legs "as if they didn't belong to me." Two years previously she began using a cane because of gait unsteadiness. One year ago she stopped driving because of an inability to feel the gas pedal and brake. Recently the numbness spread to involve her hands.

For the last year she had complained of sudden pains of 1-2 seconds duration, variable in location, but usually sharply localized to one or the other leg. She had seen several physicians, had a workup for diabetes mellitus which was negative, and received Vitamin B_{12} injections without benefit.

On examination she was a pleasant, intelligent woman. Mental status was normal. Pupils were unequal, R 3.5 mm, L 1.5 mm. The left pupil was irregular. Corrected visual acuity was 20/30 bilaterally. The right pupil reacted slowly to light and accommodation; the left pupil accommodated but did not react to light. Cranial nerves were otherwise normal. Strength was normal. She was completely areflexic in all limbs. Position and vibration perception were reduced in the arms and absent in the legs; light touch, pain, and temperature sensation was normal. Gait was grossly ataxic, broad-based, and slapping.

NEUROANATOMICAL CLUE:

Accommodation originates as a cortical (voluntary) impulse to gaze at a near object; pupilloconstriction, a local brainstem reflex, occurs with accommodation. A loss of constriction to light with preserved accommodation may occur with lesions near the aqueduct.

QUESTIONS:

1. What is the diagnosis? What is the differential diagnosis of progressive ataxia with numbness?

2. What is the significance of the pupillary abnormalities in this patient?

3. What test(s) would most help establish the diagnosis?

4. What are other CNS syndromes that occur with this disease?

5. What is the appropriate treatment?

ANSWERS:

1. Tabes dorsalis - Ataxia, areflexia (legs first), posterior-column deficits and lightening pains; also urinary incontinence, visceral crises, Argyll Robertson pupils, trophic ulcers leading to Charcot joints. Pathology includes destruction of posterior roots with secondary degeneration of posterior columns.

   Other progressive ataxias with areflexia include: a) inherited ataxias (Friedreich or Roussy-Lévy); b) chronic polyneuropathies (diabetes, alcohol, Guillain-Barré); and c) combined systems disease - B_{12} deficiency (expect pyramidal tract signs, glossitis, macrocytic anemia). The progressive inherited ataxias do not have the Argyll Robertson pupil.

2. The Argyll Robertson pupil is: a) small; b) irregular; c) reactive to accommodation (constricts); d) unreactive to light (direct or consensual). Acuity should be reasonably preserved in order to make the diagnosis. Suggestive of neurosyphilis, the Argyll Robertson pupil may also be seen in diabetes mellitus, multiple sclerosis, brainstem encephalitis, and pineal tumors. In most, but not all, instances of nonsyphilitic Argyll Robertson pupils, the pupil is normal in size and regular. A "true" Argyll Robertson pupil can be unilateral or bilateral and may respond normally to mydriatics.

3. CSF examination. Expect a) lymphocytosis, up to $5/mm^3$, b) modest elevation of protein with increased gamma globulin fraction, c) positive VDRL. With late ("burned out") neurosyphilis, CSF inflammation may be absent and VDRL may be negative; nonetheless, a CSF fluorescent treponemal antibody absorption test (FTA) should be positive, even in late cases.

4. a) Syphilitic meningitis occurs within 2 years of primary contact and is often asymptomatic. It is a necessary prerequisite for the development of late neurosyphilis.

b) <u>Meningovascular syphilis</u> usually occurs 6-15 years following initial infection; strokes occur; think of meningovascular syphilis in all young people with cerebrovascular accidents; pathology includes a panarteritis.

c) <u>Progressive optic atrophy</u> is due to perioptic meningitis.

d) <u>General paresis</u>. Symptoms begin 15-20 years after infection and consist of progressive dementia, occasionally with grandiose delusions, tremor, and seizures. Patients with general paresis usually have Argyll Robertson pupils. Consider syphilis in <u>all</u> dementia workups.

e) Apart from meningitis, few of the syndromes exist in the pure form and, in most patients, combinations are found.

5. <u>Penicillin</u> - 12 million units of aqueous crystalline PenC IV QD for 10-15 days, or 1.2-2.4 million units QD of Procaine PenG IM for 10-15 days, with 500 mg Probenecid PO Q 6 hours.

PEARLS:

1. Syphilis is the most <u>chronic CNS infection</u> of man.

2. <u>Untreated</u>, only one-third of patients with syphilitic meningitis will develop late manifestations of neurosyphilis.

3. <u>Congenital neurosyphilis</u>, acquired between months 4-7 of gestation, may take any of the adult forms or present as hydrocephalus. Hutchinson triad (dental deformities, interstitial keratitis, and deafness) may be present.

4. Preservation of the light reflex with poor accommodation to near objects ("<u>reverse Argyll Robertson pupil</u>") is frequently noted in the elderly population and occasionally following diphtheria infection.

PITFALLS:

1. Remember syphilitic meningitis as a cause of aseptic meningitis, particularly in young adults.

2. Following treatment of neurosyphilis, repeat CSF examinations every 3-6 months are mandatory until CSF clears; if pleocytosis persists 6 months after treatment, another course of penicillin is indicated.

3. Adie's pupil (tonic pupil) may be mistaken for Argyll Robertson pupil. It is seen in healthy young women and consists of a unilateral or bilateral large pupil which reacts to light, but recovers slowly to light and accommodation. In Adie's syndrome there is also areflexia at knees. Pathology probably consists of degeneration of postganglionic parasympathetic (ciliary body) neurons, innervating the iris. Do not mistake for neurosyphilis!

REFERENCES

1. Adams RD, Victor M: <u>Principles of Neurology</u>. New York, McGraw-Hill, 1982.
2. Brodal A: <u>Neurological Anatomy in Relation to Clinical Medicine</u>. 3rd edition, New York, Oxford University Press, 1981.
3. Ducas J, Robson HG: Cerebrospinal fluid penicillin levels during therapy for latent syphilis. J Am Med Assoc 246:2583, 1981.
4. Felman YM: Lumbar puncture in asymptomatic neurosyphilis. Arch Int Med 145:422, 1985.
5. Lowenfeld I: The Argyll Robertson pupil - 1869-1969: A critical survey of the literature. Surv Ophthalmol 14:199, 1969.
6. Merritt H, Adams RD, Solomon H: <u>Neurosyphilis</u>. New York, Oxford University Press, 1946.
7. Wiesel J: Lumbar puncture in asymptomatic late syphilis: an analysis of the benefits and risks. Arch Int Med 145:465, 1985.

WEAKNESS, CRAMPS, AND FASCICULATIONS

CASE 3: A 67-year-old man was admitted with a two-month history of progressive limb weakness. His illness began insidiously with weakness of the left leg associated with cramps. He began to fall frequently and noted intermittent numbness of the right leg. One month later progressive weakness of his arms began. Vision, swallowing, and bowel/bladder function were unaffected. There was no toxin exposure. Family history was negative for neurologic disease.

General examination and mentation were normal. Cranial nerves were normal except for bilateral tongue fasciculations. There were fasciculations in all extremities, most prominently in biceps, quadriceps and dorsum of hands. All muscle groups below the neck were weak, and in the upper extremities there was atrophy of biceps, triceps, and intrinsic muscles of the hands. Gait was unstable, slow, and on a broad base. Tone was increased in the legs; all reflexes were hyperactive (including jawjerk) and there were bilateral extensor plantar responses. Sensation, despite his complaint of numbness, was intact to all modalities.

QUESTIONS:

1. What is the significance of fasciculations and how do they differ from fibrillations? What other portions of the nervous system are involved in this patient?

2. A CSF exam was normal. EMG revealed normal nerve conduction velocity, fibrillation potentials, and giant motor unit potentials. What other tests might you suggest?

3. What is the most likely diagnosis?

4. What treatments are available?

5. What is the prognosis?

NEUROANATOMICAL CLUE:

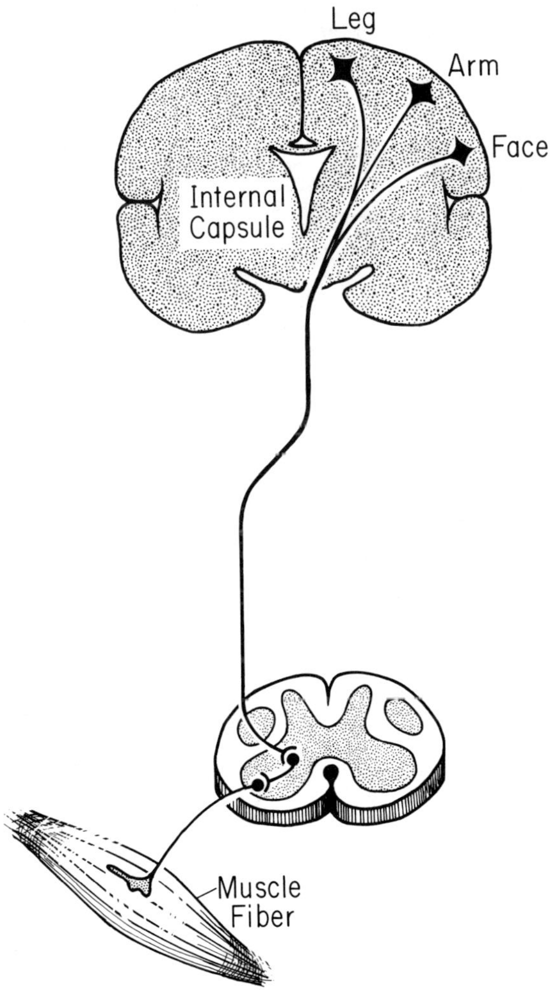

ANSWERS:

1. Fasciculations result from the spontaneous firing of a motor unit, i.e., a motor nerve and the muscle fibers that it innervates. Fibrillations result from contraction of a single denervated muscle fiber. Fasciculations are common in diseases of the anterior horn cell or ventral root. Hyperreflexia and extensor plantars indicate lesions of upper motor neurons. Thus, the clinical picture suggests a lower motor neuron lesion, manifested by atrophy, fasciculations, and fibrillations, and an upper motor neuron lesion, manifested by spasticity and bilateral Babinskis. Neuroanatomical clue shows a diagram of the motor system.

2. The absence of sensory loss and presence of fasciculations in the legs makes syringomyelia or other cervical cord lesions (disc, tumor) unlikely. Myelography of the cervical canal and foramen magnum region, with post-myelogram CT scan of the area is advisable in all questionable cases.

3. Amyotrophic lateral sclerosis (ALS). ALS usually presents between the ages 40-60, although onset as early as adolescence and as late as the 8th decade may occur. Normal CSF rules out enterovirus infection (e.g., polio) or syphilitic amyotrophy. ALS typically involves both upper and lower motor neurons; involvement of only upper motor neurons (primary lateral sclerosis), lower motor neurons (progressive amyotrophy), or bulbar motor neurons (progressive bulbar palsy) may occur.

4. The pathogenesis is unknown and no specific treatments (save symptomatic) exist. No convincing evidence of viral infection has been found. Raised levels of heavy metals in the spinal cord of ALS patients have been found, but the significance of this finding is unknown. Plasmapheresis, chemotherapy, transfer factor, gangliosides, and snake venom have been given to ALS patients without benefit. Recently, investigators have treated patients with thyrotropic releasing hormone.

5. Fifty percent of ALS patients are dead within 3 years of diagnosis. Twenty percent of patients are alive at 5 years, and rarely, remissions have been reported.

PEARLS:

1. Other symptoms of ALS: a) muscle cramps - common; b) sensory complaints, usually mild, in 25% of patients; c) emotional lability due to corticobulbar disease.

2. Epidemiology: increased incidence of antecedent trauma and polio in ALS patients; disease is more common in males than females.

3. Uncommon variants of anterior horn cell disease include: a) Werdnig-Hoffmann disease - age of onset is from neonatal period to childhood; b) Kugelberg-Welander disease - adolescent onset, proximal limbs involved early; c) "Familial ALS" - autosomal dominant, usually affects young adults.

4. Recent studies have demonstrated that motorneuron-specific growth factors are produced in muscle; the possible importance of these factors in the pathogenesis of ALS is currently under active study.

PITFALLS:

1. Do not diagnose ALS unless weakness is present. Chronic fasciculations without weakness, sometimes with associated cramping, are common, especially in athletes and medical personnel, and are benign.

2. Question the diagnosis of ALS if early symptoms suggest extraocular muscle or bowel/bladder involvement, or if there is any objective sensory loss.

REFERENCES

1. Gurney ME, Belton AC, Cashman N, Antel JP: Inhibition of terminal axonal sprouting by serum from patients with amyotrophic lateral sclerosis. N Engl J Med 311:933, 1984.
2. Hudson AJ: Amyotrophic lateral sclerosis and its association with dementia, parkinsonism, and other neurological disorders: a review. Brain 104:217, 1981.
3. Kurtzke JF, Beefe GW: Epidemiology of amyotrophic lateral sclerosis: 1. A case-control comparison based on ALS deaths. Neurology 30:453, 1980.
4. Mulder DW, Howard FM Jr: Patient resistance and prognosis in amyotrophic lateral sclerosis. Mayo Clin Proc 51:537, 1976.

UNSTEADINESS OF GAIT AND BARKING

CASE 4: A 53-year-old man complained of intermittent blurred vision followed 1 month later by vertigo and an unstable gait. His medical history was remarkable only for mild hypertension well controlled with diuretics. Examination revealed convergence-retraction nystagmus, spontaneous upbeat nystagmus, left palatal weakness, mild limb incoordination, and gait ataxia. Mental status was normal. CT scan and LP (including gamma globulin and VDRL) were normal. EEG showed shifting frontotemporal slowing. No cause for his symptoms could be found, and he was discharged only to be readmitted three weeks later because of further gait unsteadiness. In addition, his wife noted a flattening of affect, decrease in intellectual function, and slowing of speech. Mental status testing now revealed that serial tasks were performed slowly and recent memory was poor. During the next week he became progressively abulic, emotionally labile, and exhibited unusual posturing of his hands. Grasp and snout responses were now present. He startled staff by barking, growling, or meowing when they entered the room. A repeat EEG was obtained and is shown below:

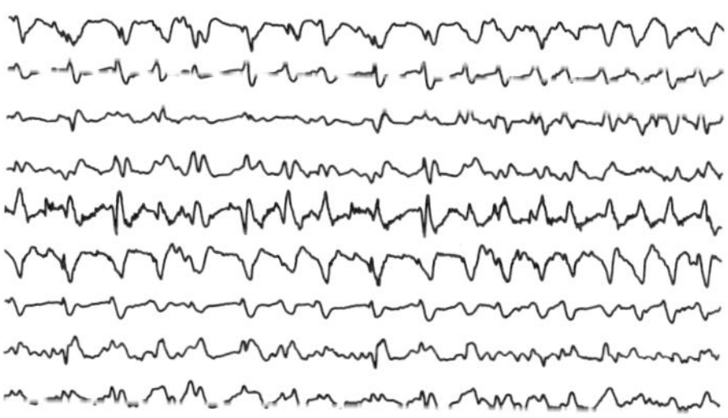

QUESTIONS:

1. What is the significance of the EEG abnormality?

2. What is the cause of this man's disease?

3. What other diseases have a similar cause?

4. What is the usual clinical course?

5. Is there evidence for transmissibility of this disease in man?

ANSWERS:

1. High voltage synchronous sharp waves superimposed on low voltage background is characteristic of subacute spongiform encephalopathy, also known as Creutzfeldt-Jakob (C-J) disease.

2. "Slow Virus" - Infectious etiology by an as yet unidentified transmissible agent. The agent is not a classic virus and cannot be visualized under the electron microscope or be neutralized by antibody. The disease can be transferred from man to chimpanzee by intracerebral inoculation.

3. Kuru, which occurs in the Fore tribe in New Guinea, is a rapidly (3-6 month) evolving ataxia followed by global mental deficits and death and is transmitted by cannibalism. There are two animal examples of transmissible spongiform encephalopathy: scrapie (sheep) and transmissible mink encephalopathy.

4. The clinical course is divided into the prodromal and dementing myoclonic phases. During prodrome, behavioral changes, subtle intellectual decline, and visual symptoms are common. The disease is usually fatal within 1 year from onset.

5. Several cases of human-to-human transmission are known, including two via contaminated electrodes inserted into brain and one via corneal transplantation. In addition, patients with Creutzfeldt-Jakob disease have an increased incidence of having had brain and ocular surgery within 2 years preceding the onset of symptoms.

PEARLS:

1. The myoclonus of Creutzfeldt-Jakob disease typically includes individual twitches of small, distal, limb muscles. Nearly all patients develop myoclonus at some time during their illness. An exaggerated startle response is another form of myoclonus that may occur with Creutzfeldt-Jakob disease.

2. The pathology of Creutzfeldt-Jakob disease consists of spongiform changes within gray matter which are small round or oval vacuoles in the neuropil and are

pathognomonic. These changes are not to be confused with _status spongiosus_, which consists of gliosis with cavitory lesions in gray matter and is nonspecific. Spongiform changes may not be present in cases of long duration prior to death.

3. Creutzfeldt-Jakob disease is usually a disease of _late middle age_, although cases between age 27 and 80 have been reported.

4. Fifteen percent of cases have at least one other affected _family_ member, and several geographic clusterings have been reported.

PITFALLS:

1. _Tissues and fluids from patients with unexplained dementias should be handled cautiously_. High titers of the Creutzfeldt-Jakob agent are present in brain and spinal cord and low titers in CSF, lymph nodes, spleen, liver, lung, kidney, and cornea. There is no evidence thus far that stool, urine, or saliva is infectious, and no special precautions have been advised. Blood specimens should be handled as potentially infectious.

2. _Not all myoclonic dementias are Creutzfeldt-Jakob in origin_. Alzheimer's disease may evolve rapidly and include myoclonus. Other rare causes of myoclonic dementia are adult lipidosis (Kuf's type) and subacute sclerosing panencephalitis (SSPE) which is due to a chronic measles virus infection in brain.

REFERENCES

1. Bockman JM, Kingsbury DT, McKinley MP, Bendheim PE, Prusiner SB: Creutzfeldt-Jakob disease prior proteins in human brains. N Engl J Med 312:73, 1985.
2. Gajdusek DC, Gibbs CJ Jr, Asher DM, et al: Precautions in medical care of, and in handling materials from patients with transmissible virus dementia (Creutzfeldt-Jakob Disease). N Engl J Med 297:1253, 1977.
3. Kimberlin RH: Scrapie: the disease and the infectious agent. Trends Neurosci 7:312, 1984.
4. Masters CL, Richardson EP Jr: Subacute spongiform encephalopathy (Creutzfeldt-Jakob Disease): The nature and progression of spongiform change. Brain 101:333, 1978.

HEADACHE AND PROGRESSIVE HEMIPARESIS

CASE 5: A 55-year-old woman with known hypertension had the sudden onset at work of weakness of her right leg, then weakness of her right arm and difficulty speaking. She had complained for the past 3 days of headache, which worsened that morning. She had stopped taking her blood pressure medication 2 months previously because she was "feeling well." Her weakness progressed over the next half hour and she was taken to the emergency room where she was found to have a blood pressure of 240/140. She was alert but aphasic; had a right visual field defect, right facial weakness, hemiparesis, and right extensor plantar response. She became nauseated and vomited.

NEUROANATOMICAL CLUE:

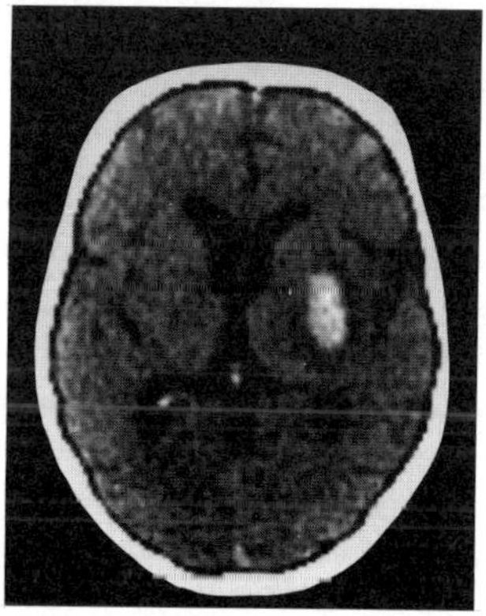

QUESTIONS:

1. What is the nature and location of this lesion?
2. What is the underlying vascular pathology?
3. What is the appropriate treatment?
4. What are the reasons for deterioration in this group of patients?
5. What is the prognosis for intracerebral hemorrhage?

ANSWERS:

1. Intracerebral hemorrhage - left putamen.

2. Small vessel disease - arteriolar disruption due to hypertension (nearly always present). Other less common causes include bleeding from a vascular malformation, tumor, a hemorrhagic disorder, and vasculitis.

3. Lower blood pressure, give steroids (Dexamethasone, 10 mg bolus, then 4 mg q.i.d.) and, because of drowsiness, give mannitol 1-2 gm/kg/IV, or glycerol. There is no convincing evidence for improved prognosis with surgery for deep intracerebral hemorrhage. This patient stabilized after 24 hours and made a full recovery.

4. With large bleeds, herniation (uncal or central) occurs. Deterioration from the intracranial hemorrhage itself generally evolves within 6 hours. Later deterioration usually is due to the effects of mass and/or edema, not rebleeding.

5. The overall mortality from intracerebral hemorrhage is 30%, but for those patients in coma it is more than 95%. With prompt diagnosis and early treatment, these figures can probably be improved.

PEARLS:

1. Headache is usually, but not always, present in intracerebral hemorrhage; headache may also be present in other stroke syndromes (especially embolism).

2. CT scan distinguishes cerebral hemorrhage from infarct. Virtually all hemorrhages are positive on CT scan.

PITFALLS:

1. Small putaminal hemorrhage may present as pure motor hemiparesis, mimicking a lacunar stroke. Thus, do not anticoagulate small "embolic" strokes or transient ischemic attacks before doing a CT scan to be certain that the patient does not have a small hemorrhage.

2. CSF may be normal with small putaminal hemorrhage.

REFERENCES

1. Herbstein DJ, Schaumberg HH: Hypertensive intracerebral hematoma: An investigation of the initial hemorrhage and rebleeding using chromium labeled erythrocytes. Arch Neurol 30:412, 1974.
2. Hier DB, Davis KR, Richardson EP Jr, Mohr JP: Hypertensive putaminal hemorrhage. Ann Neurol 1:152, 1977.
3. Kase CS: Lobar intracerebral hematomas: Clinical and CT analysis of 22 cases. Neurology 32:1146, 1982.
4. Mohr JP, Kase C, Adams RD: Cerebrovascular diseases. In _Harrison's Principles of Internal Medicine_, McGraw-Hill, New York, 1983.
5. Nath FP: Prognosis in intracerebral hemorrhage. Acta Neurochir 67:29, 1983.
6. Ojemann RG, Mohr JP: Hypertensive brain hemorrhage. Clin Neurosurg 23:220, 1976.
7. Portenoy RK, Abissi CJ, Lipton RB, et al: Headache in cerebrovascular disease. Stroke 15:1009, 1984.
8. Sandercock P, Molyneux A, Warlow C: Value of comuted tomography in patients with stroke. Oxfordshire Community Stroke Project 290:193, 1985.

"PURE" MOTOR STROKE

CASE 6: A 62-year-old married brewmaster at a local brewery, awoke one morning with a right hemiplegia. There was no associated headache, visual loss, or sensory loss. He was able to speak to his wife normally. Two years previously, he was found to have a blood pressure of 180/110, but was treated with antihypertensives for only 6 months. He tastes beer each day at work.

Examination: BP 160/100, pulse 72 and regular; normal carotid and cardiac exam; fluent speech, normal reading, writing, naming and repetition; a right hemiplegia, face = arm = leg; normal sensation, right hyperreflexia, and a right extensor plantar response.

NEUROANATOMICAL CLUE: Horizontal Section Through the Internal Capsule

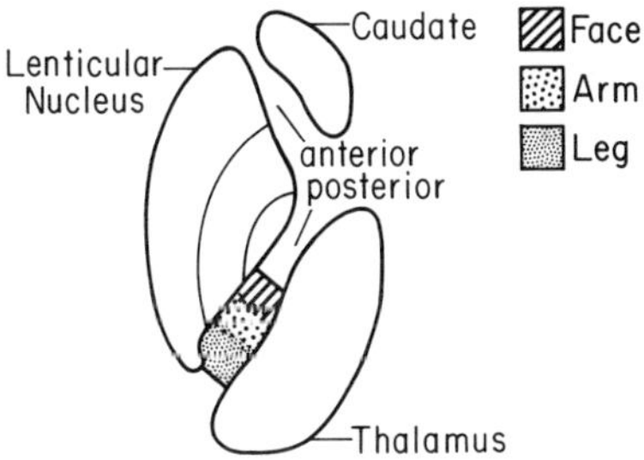

QUESTIONS:

1. What was the first clue that this patient did not have a "typical" stroke with right-sided paralysis?

2. What is the differential diagnosis?

3. What tests would be helpful to establish the correct diagnosis?

4. What is the predisposing, treatable factor for his stroke?

5. How should the patient now be treated?

6. What is the prognosis for recovery?

ANSWERS:

1. In right-handed persons with acute strokes, a right hemiplegia (involving face, arm, and leg) without sensory loss or aphasia is due to a subcortical lesion. Middle cerebral artery occlusion would not produce a pure motor deficit.

2. A lacunar infarction in the posterior limb of the left internal capsule or in the left pons is the most likely diagnosis. A small hemorrhage in a similar location is also possible. Rarely, a cerebral metastasis could present in this way.

3. An EEG should be normal; A CT scan should be either normal or show a small area of decreased density in basal ganglia (internal capsule area) or pons, establishing a diagnosis of small vessel subcortical (lacunar) infarction.

4. Hypertension. Adequate control of blood pressure will reduce the risk of lacunar infarction, as well as that of intracerebral hemorrhage.

5. Conservative management, including physical therapy. Do not lower blood pressure acutely, as hypertensive patients may required increased blood pressure to maintain cerebral blood flow. Anticoagulants are not indicated.

6. Good; physical therapy may help to speed recovery.

PEARLS:

1. Patients with hemiplegia of cortical origin usually cannot give a clear and coherent history, as they have cognitive loss secondary to their cortical infarction.

2. Pure motor hemiplegia, pure sensory stroke, "clumsy-hand" dysarthria, and ataxia-crural paresis are classic lacunar syndromes.

3. Hypertension is the most important preventable risk factor of stroke and treatment of hypertension may be the reason for the declining incidence of stroke in recent years.

4. The vascular lesions responsible for both lacunar strokes and hemorrhagic strokes consist of hyaline degeneration of arterioles.

PITFALLS:

1. Patients with pure motor hemiplegia, particularly with lesions of the left internal capsule, may have dysarthria or a non-fluent aphasia, usually transient.

2. Pure motor deficits that do not involve face, arm, and leg may be due to anterior or middle cerebral artery infarction and should not be assumed to be lacunar. Remember, large vessel infarcts have a different pathogenesis and treatment.

3. Rarely, a lenticulostriate embolus from a distant site (heart or carotids) or from atherosclerosis at the origin (stem) of the middle cerebral artery can produce capsular, e.g., pure motor, infarction. Not all small vessel strokes are lacunar.

REFERENCES

1. Fisher CM: A lacunar stroke. The dysarthria-clumsy hand syndrome. Neurology 17:614, 1967.
2. Fisher CM: Ataxic hemiparesis. A pathologic study. Arch Neurol 35:126, 1978.
3. Fisher CM: Thalamic pure sensory stroke: a pathologic study. Neurology 28:1141, 1978.
4. Fisher CM: Capsular infarcts. The underlying vascular lesions. Arch Neurol 36:65, 1979.
5. Huang CY, Lui FS: Ataxic hemiparesis, localization and clinical features. Stroke 15:363, 1984.
6. Mohr JP: Lacunar infarcts. Stroke 13:3, 1982.
7. Santamaria J: Cerebral infarction of the basal ganglia due to embolism from the heart. Stroke 14:911, 1983.
8. Weisberg LA: Lacunar infarcts. Clinical and computed tomographic correlations. Arch Neurol 39:37, 1982.
9. Whisnant JP: The decline of stroke. Stroke 15:160, 1984.

STROKE WITH APHASIA AND SEIZURES

CASE 7: A 51-year-old engineer developed fatigue, chills, low grade fever, right shoulder pain and then had a syncopal episode. Blood gases revealed hypoxemia and respiratory alkalosis. A lung scan showed evidence of pulmonary emboli. He was treated with intravenous heparin. Two days later, his wife noted his neck and face had become red; there was sudden dyspnea, then inability to speak, and a right hemiplegia. Examination demonstrated an aphasia which was characterized by little spontaneous speech but good comprehension. Reading and writing were impaired. A CT scan performed on the day of the stroke was normal. An EEG showed focal slowing in the left frontal area. One month later he developed right-sided motor seizures which were controlled with phenytoin.

NEUROANATOMICAL CLUE:

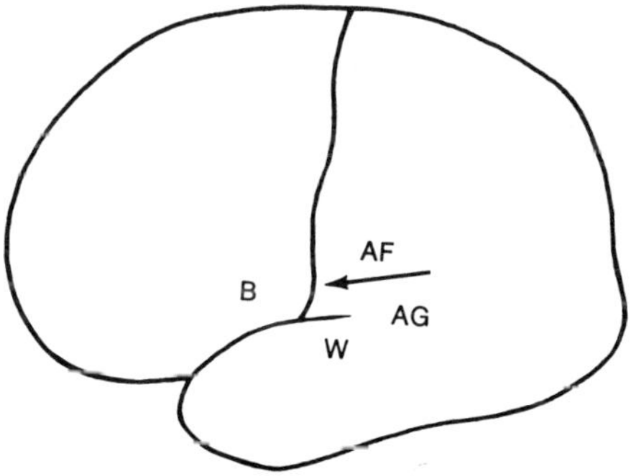

QUESTIONS:

1. What is the connection between the patient's pulmonary embolism and his stroke?

2. How might the seizure be explained?

3. Why was spontaneous speech so sparse while comprehension was so good?

4. Is it likely that hypotension or hypoxemia would produce a specific aphasic syndrome? Why or why not?

5. What is the appropriate treatment for this stroke?

ANSWERS:

1. Recurrent pulmonary emboli - sudden increase in right atrial pressure - paradoxical embolus through a patent foramen ovale.

2. Seizures occur in approximately 10% of embolic strokes, probably because emboli lodge distally in the brain and produce cortical infarcts; seizures rarely occur following cerebral thrombosis.

3. The patient had non-fluent or Broca's aphasia, which is characterized by sparse stuttering speech, relatively preserved comprehension, and impaired repetition and naming. A right hemiplegia often co-exists.

   Neuroanatomical clue: the perisylvian speech area. Speech production involves 4 regions in this area moving from posterior to anterior: Wernicke's area (W), the angular gyrus (AG), the arcuate fasciculus (AF), and Broca's area (B).

4. No. Acute metabolic insults produce generalized cerebral disturbances with clouding of consciousness. Focal symptoms may occur in some patients, particularly with hypoglycemia or with a metabolic disturbance superimposed on preexisting cerebrovascular disease, but aphasias are rare in hypoxemia or hypotension.

5. Unless the source of embolism can be eliminated long-term anticoagulation is indicated. Surgical venous ligation may be necessary in patients with recurrent pulmonary or cerebral emboli due to peripheral vascular disease.

PEARLS

1. A quick aphasia test: reading, writing, repetition, and naming.

2. In dysarthria the words are unclear - in aphasia, the words are usually wrong.

3. Patients with Broca's aphasia are unable to write with either hand.

4. Stroke syndromes of aphasia without hemiparesis or stroke with seizure: Think of embolus.

5. There are two types of Broca's aphasia:

   "Big Broca" - Some difficulty with spoken and written language, protracted mutism and hemiplegia; due to widespread infarction of inferior frontal lobe, poor prognosis for the aphasia.
   "Baby Broca" - Comprehension of speech and writing normal or nearly so; dysphasia rapidly improves; restricted infarction of inferior frontal lobule (Broca's area); excellent prognosis.

6. In general, conduction and Broca aphasias have the best prognosis; global aphasias with marked impairment of expression and comprehension have the worst prognosis. Left-handedness is a favorable prognostic sign, as is the absence of a hemiparesis.

PITFALLS

1. The acute onset of aphasia without hemiparesis (e.g., after cardiac catheterization) is often misinterpreted as being due to a psychiatric cause. Embolism to a middle cerebral branch is usually responsible. Paraphasic errors are usually the clue to the presence of aphasia.

2. Think of the possibility of paradoxical cerebral embolism in any patient with cerebral embolus without a carotid lesion or cardiac source, particularly in patients with enhanced potential for venous thrombosis. Preexisting pulmonary emboli or venous thromboses are frequently clinically silent at the time of the stroke.

FOLLOW-UP:

A repeat CT scan 1 month after this patient's stroke demonstrated a left frontal lobe infarction.

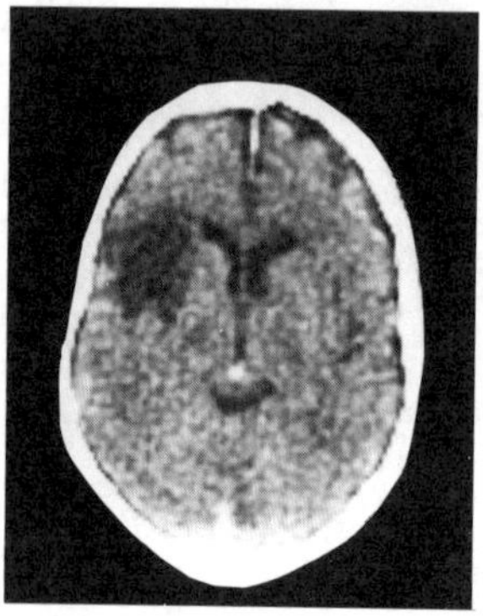

REFERENCES

1. Benson DF, Geschwind N: The aphasias and related disturbances. In Clinical Neurology, Hagerstown, MD, Harper and Row, 1983.
2. Cerebral Embolism Study Group: Immediate anticoagulation of embolic stroke: brain hemorrhage and management options. Stroke 15:779, 1984.
3. Jones HR, Caplan LR, et al.: Cerebral emboli of paradoxical origin. Ann Neurol 13:314, 1983.
4. Kertesz A, McCabe P: Recovery patterns and prognosis in aphasia. Brain 100:1, 1977.
5. McNeil MR: Current concepts in adult aphasia. Int Rehab Med 6:128, 1984.
6. Mohr JP, et al.: Broca's aphasia: Pathologic and clinical. Neurology 28:311, 1979.
7. Naeser MA, Hayward RW: Lesion localization in aphasia with cranial computed tomography and the Boston Diagnostic aphasia exam. Neurology 28:545, 1978.
8. Shields RW Jr, Lavreno R, Lachman T, Victor M: Anticoagulant-related hemorrhage in acute cerebral embolism. Stroke 15:425, 1984.

HEADACHE, FATIGUE, AND SUDDEN BLINDNESS

CASE 8: A 73-year-old man awoke with complete blindness in his right eye. For the past month he had complained of severe constant frontal headache, beginning on the right, but rapidly becoming bilateral. In addition, fatigue and anorexia appeared at about the same time. One day earlier, he noted a brief (less than 15 minute) episode of "darkening" of vision in his right eye.

On examination, the right pupil reacted to consensual but not to direct light. There was no light perception in the right eye. The right optic nerve head was swollen and pale; several small linear hemorrhages were present. Remainder of neurologic exam was normal.

QUESTIONS:

1. What is the diagnosis?

2. What are the characteristic findings on facial artery palpation in this disease?

3. What single laboratory test would be most helpful in support of your diagnosis?

4. How is a definitive diagnosis made?

5. What is the significance of this patient's weight loss and fatigue?

6. What is the appropriate therapy? How long should it be continued?

ANSWERS:

1. Giant cell or temporal arteritis.

2. Pain, thickening, and decreased pulsation of one or more vessels is characteristic.

3. Erythrocyte sedimentation rate (ESR) - elevated in more than 95% of patients.

4. Temporal artery biopsy - granulomatous inflammation of the vessel wall, often with secondary thrombosis: diagnostic of giant cell (temporal) arteritis.

5. Systemic symptoms, including fever, anorexia, fatigue and anemia are often present in giant cell arteritis; polymyalgia rheumatica may be present.

6. Steroid therapy should be started immediately in patients with suspected giant cell arteritis and visual symptoms. Initially, 60 mg of prednisone or its equivalent daily, with a very slow taper titrated to patient's symptoms and ESR. Prolonged therapy (more than 6 months) is effective in preventing blindness and reducing systemic symptoms.

   //Partial or complete visual loss occurs in over 50% of untreated patients with giant cell arteritis; following monocular blindness, loss of vision in the second eye may develop rapidly//

PEARLS:

1. One or two days of steroid therapy will not affect biopsy pathology. Steroids should be instituted while arrangements are made for biopsy.

2. Difficulty combing and brushing hair, due to tenderness of involved vessels or to scalp ischemia, may be present. Jaw claudication may sometimes occur.

3. Frequently, visual loss may be out of proportion to changes on fundoscopy. Typical fundoscopic abnormalities include disc swelling, pallor, narrowing of retinal arterioles and linear (nerve fiber) hemorrhages. In some patients, central retinal artery occlusion is present.

4. Although generally considered a disease of the external carotid system, this is not always the case, and generalized large-vessel arteritis may be present. In untreated cases, stroke and myocardial infarction due to arteritis are frequent causes of death.

5. Temporal arteritis is usually a disease of late life, although typical giant cell arteritis does occasionally occur in young people as well.

PITFALLS:

1. Think of giant cell arteritis in all elderly persons with unexplained headache, visual difficulties, or the recent development of systemic symptoms.

2. Palpation of the superficial temporal artery alone will not disclose abnormalities in the majority of patients; a complete facial artery exam should be performed in patients with suspected giant cell arteritis.

3. Arteritis is typically segmental, with diseased areas interspersed with regions of normal vessel wall. A negative biopsy, therefore, does not exclude the diagnosis, and several biopsies may be required.

REFERENCES

1. Cull RE: Internal carotid artery occlusion caused by giant cell arteritis. J Neurol Neurosurg Psychiat 42:1066, 1979.
2. Goodman BW Jr: Temporal arteritis. Am J Med 67:839, 1979.
3. Hall S, Hunder GG: Is temporal artery biopsy prudent? Mayo Clin Proc 59:790, 1984.
4. Hall S, Lie JT, Kurland LT, Persellin S, O'Brien PC, Hunder GG: The therapeutic impact of temporal artery biopsy. Lancet 2:1217, 1983.
5. Hamilton CR, Shelly WM, Tumulty PA: Giant cell arteritis. Medicine (Baltimore) 50:1, 1971.
6. Huston KA, Hunder GG, Lie TJ et al: Temporal arteritis. A 25 year epidemiologic, clinical, pathologic study. Ann Int Med 88:162, 1978.
7. Walsh and Hoyt: Clinical Neuro-Ophthalmology, Baltimore, Williams & Wilkins, pp. 1878-1886, 1969.

TRANSIENT APHASIA AND VISUAL LOSS

CASE 9: A 53-year-old man with a history of a myocardial infarction 2 years previously came to his physician because of an episode of clumsiness of his right hand. The episode occurred while eating dinner and forced him to use his left hand. There were no associated symptoms, and the clumsiness disappeared over the course of 1 hour. On questioning by his physician, the patient reported two other episodes that had occurred in the past 3 months. In one, which began abruptly during a conversation at a cocktail party, the patient had difficulty using words. His wife thought he was drunk because he was using the wrong words in sentences and didn't understand fully when she spoke to him. In a few minutes he had returned to normal. The second episode was a period of transient blindness when the patient noticed a "shade" coming down over his left eye. On examination: BP 150/90, pulse regular. There were no carotid bruits. Neurologic examination was normal.

QUESTIONS:

1. This patient had a transient ischemic attack (TIA). In what vascular territory did the TIA occur?
2. What is the probable mechanism?
3. What feature(s) characterize TIAs from a cardiac source?
4. What percentage of patients with TIAs will have a stroke?
5. What should the workup involve?
6. What is the most appropriate treatment in this patient?

NEUROANATOMICAL CLUE:

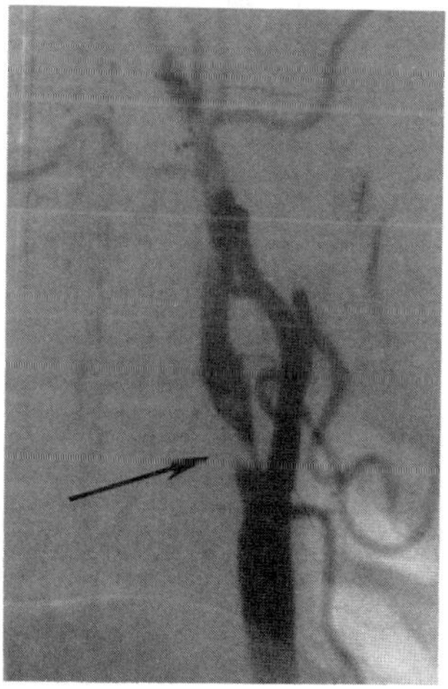

ANSWERS:

1. All three TIAs were in the <u>left anterior circulation</u> (carotid artery) territory.

2. Up to 80% of patients with TIA have <u>atherosclerotic disease</u> (stenosis or ulceration) of the artery appropriate to their symptoms. The TIAs themselves are presumably due to microemboli or hemodynamic changes distal to the diseased segment.

3. Cardiac emboli typically produce <u>TIAs in more than one large vessel territory</u> (e.g., right and left carotid, carotid and vertebrobasilar), show rapid resolution of neurological deficit, and may produce seizures or transient loss of consciousness at onset of stroke.

4. In most reports, approximately <u>one-third</u> of patients with untreated TIAs will subsequently develop stroke within 3 years. The risk is highest in the year following the TIA.

5. If facilities are available, <u>bilateral carotid arteriography</u> should be performed. Careful cardiac evaluation, including at least auscultation and EKG to rule out valvular disease or arrhythmia, should precede angiography. Cardiac echo and Holter monitor are are indicated where suspicion of valvular disease or arrhythmia is high and are especially important in younger patients with TIA, who have a lower likelihood of carotid disease.

6. If the angiogram demonstrates significant stenosis or an ulcerated plaque in the left extracranial carotid system, <u>surgery</u> (endarterectomy) is indicated. If the angiogram is normal or a lesion is present but is surgically inaccessible, <u>antiplatelet drugs</u> are the treatment of choice, followed by <u>anticoagulation</u> if the patient fails antiplatelet drugs.

PEARLS

1. <u>Examination of facial pulses in TIAs</u>.

   The supraorbital artery, located beneath the medial aspect of the upper eyelid, is a branch of the ophthalmic artery and is fed from the ipsilateral internal carotid; the superficial temporal artery, which lies anterior to the ear, is supplied by the external carotid system. In normal circumstances, external compression of the superficial temporal artery will result in no change in the supraorbital pulse. In acute internal carotid occlusion, however, the supraorbital pulse will disappear with superficial temporal compression due to reversal of flow in the supraorbital artery, which is now supplied by the external carotid circulation.

2. In the recently completed Canadian Cooperative Study of TIA, <u>aspirin</u> was found to be effective in preventing stroke in men who had had a TIA within 3 months of commencing therapy. A protective effect of aspirin was not seen in women.

3. TIAs of <u>small vessel</u> origin are usually <u>stereotyped</u>; TIAs of <u>large vessel</u> origin frequently <u>vary</u> in their presentation.

PITFALLS

1. <u>Focal seizures</u> or <u>migraine</u> may produce transient neurological symptoms and mimic TIAs.

2. <u>Anemia</u>, <u>polycythemia</u>, <u>paraproteinemia</u>, and <u>thrombocytosis</u> may also be associated with TIAs and should not be overlooked.

3. Think of <u>arrhythmia</u> as a cause of TIAs.

4. <u>Significant headache</u> is usually not associated with TIAs.

REFERENCES

1. Adams HP Jr, Kassell NF, Mazuz H: The patient with TIAs. Is this the time for a new approach? Stroke 15:371, 1984.
2. Canadian Cooperative Study Group: Randomized trial of aspirin and sulfinpyrazone in threatened stroke. N Engl J Med 299:53, 1978.
3. Harrison MJG, Marshall J: Atrial fibrillation, TIAs, and completed stroke. Stroke 15:441, 1984.
4. Kistler JP, Ropper AH, Heros RC: Therapy of ischemic cerebral vascular disease due to atherothrombosis. N Engl J Med 311:27(Part 1), 311:100(Part 2), 1984.
5. Milikan CH, McDowell FH: Treatment of transient ischemic attacks. Stroke 9:299, 1978.
6. Pessin MS, et al: Clinical and angiographic features of carotid transient ischemic attacks. N Engl J Med 296:358, 1977.
7. Ross-Russell RW: Pathogenesis of transient ischemic attacks. Neurol Clin 1(1):279, 1983.
8. Wiebers DO, et al: Reversible ischemic neurologic deficit (RIND) in a community: Rochester Minn 1955-1974. Neurology 32:459, 1982.

NUMBNESS AND WEAKNESS OF ALL FOUR EXTREMITIES

<u>CASE 10</u>: A 29-year-old man developed low back pain not associated with radiation into his legs. The next day "tingling" of his fingers and toes appeared and the back pain had diminished. Two days later he noted left facial numbness and difficulty speaking and eating, and the following day he awoke with an unstable gait. Three weeks earlier he had an illness characterized by sore throat, fever, and myalgia of several days' duration.

On examination there was a severe facial diplegia and orbicularis oculi were weak bilaterally. Eye movements were normal. There was a moderate weakness of all extremities, more marked proximally. There was impaired position, vibration, and 2 point discrimination sensation in the feet, more pronounced on the left side. Sensation to pin and light touch were normal. Reflexes were absent in the lower extremities; in the upper extremities, a 1+ biceps jerk was the only deep tendon reflex elicited.

NEUROANATOMICAL CLUE:

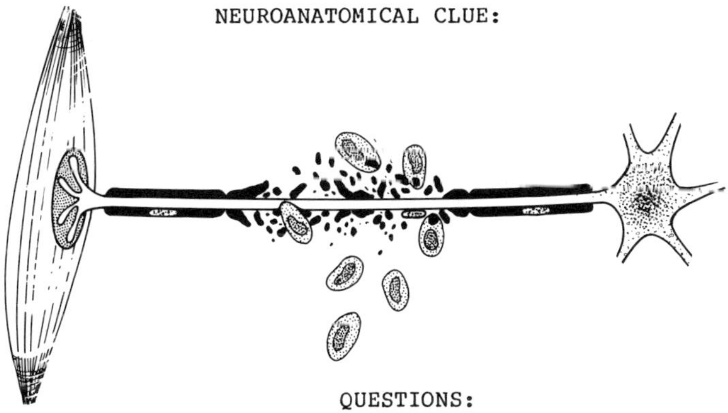

QUESTIONS:

1. What is the significance of this patient's absent reflexes?

2. What is the most likely diagnosis and what is the differential diagnosis in this patient?

3. What is the relationship of the previous upper respiratory infection to this patient's disease?

4. What is the likely etiology of this disease?

5. What is the appropriate treatment? Prognosis?

ANSWERS:

1. Bilateral, symmetrical areflexia usually signifies NEUROPATHY. In primary muscle disease, reflexes diminish only in proportion to weakness.

2. Acute idiopathic polyneuritis or Guillain Barré syndrome (GBS) is the most likely diagnosis. Other causes of acute polyneuropathy are rare, and include diphtheria (nasal voice, dysphagia, numb lips, blurred vision, antecedent sore throat), porphyria (abdominal pain, psychosis, seizures), polyarteritis nodosa (eosinophilia, elevated sedimentation rate) and toxins (triorthocresylphosphate, thallium poisoning).

3. In most patients with GBS, a viral or other infection precedes the neurologic illness. GBS followed swine flu immunization in 1976.

4. Autoimmune attack against peripheral nerve myelin. By electron microscopy, macrophage stripping of myelin lamellae can be seen. Humoral factors also play a role. Neuroanatomical clue demonstrates peripheral myelin sheath being destroyed by mononuclear cells.

5. Symptomatic. Hospitalization; close attention to respiratory status. In two controlled studies of steroid treatment, neither showed significant benefit. A national cooperative study has shown that plasmapheresis shortens the duration of mechanical ventilatory assistance needed in severe cases and should probably be given to patients who are rapidly deteriorating, preferably before they need ventilatory assistance. Prognosis is good - greater than 95% of patients make a complete recovery, although as long as 1 year may be required. Relapsing disease may occur in 5% of patients; steroids are usually effective in relapsing GBS.

PEARLS:

1. Fisher syndrome is a variant of GBS and includes ataxia, areflexia, and ophthalmoplegia.

2. The CSF in GBS is typically acellular, with increasing protein as the disease progresses (albuminocytologic dissociation). Nerve conduction velocities are slowed without signs of denervation on EMG (typical of demyelinative neuropathy).

3. GBS may occur in patients with Hodgkin's disease or following surgery. Remember, the differential diagnosis of postoperative limb weakness includes GBS, hypophosphatemia and spinal cord infarction.

4. Experimental allergic neuritis (EAN) is an animal model of GBS, induced by injection of peripheral nerve homogenate in Freund's adjuvant. The P2 protein is the major peripheral nerve protein responsible for EAN.

PITFALLS:

1. The most important cause of death in GBS is respiratory failure. It may occur with little warning; careful monitoring of vital capacity essential in early stages of disease.

2. Autonomic dysfunction may occur, occasionally dominating the syndrome, with tachycardia, labile blood pressure, loss of sweating, or episodic diaphoresis. Arrhythmias may occur and can be life threatening.

3. CSF protein may be normal in the first few days of GBS.

4. In general, neuropathies give distal weakness and myopathies give proximal weakness. GBS is one of the few neuropathies that may present with proximal weakness.

REFERENCES

1. Asbury AK, Arnason BG, Adams RD: The inflammatory lesion in idiopathic polyneuritis. Its role in pathogenesis. Medicine (Baltimore) 48:173, 1969. (The definitive pathologic study.)
2. Fisher M: An unusual variant of acute idiopathic polyneuritis (syndrome of ophthalmoplegia, ataxia and areflexia. N Engl J Med 255:57, 1956.
3. Gracey DR, et al: Respiratory failure in Guillain-Barré syndrome: A 6-year experience. Mayo Clin Proc 57(12):742. 1982.
4. Hughes RAC, Newsom-Davis JM, Perkin GD, Pierce JM. Controlled trial of prednisolone in acute polyneuropathy. Lancet 2:750, 1978. (Conclusions: Group treated with prednisone did less well than controls.)
5. Koski CL: Guillain-Barré syndrome. Neurol Clin 2(2):355, 1984.
6. Langmuir AD, Bregman DJ, Kurland LT, et al: An epidemiological and clinical evaluation of Guillain-Barré syndrome reported in association with administration of swine influenza vaccines. Am J Epidemiol 119:841, 1984.
7. Rostami A, Brown MJ, Lisak RP, Sumner AJ, Zweiman B, Pleasure DE: The role of myelin P_2 protein in the production of experimental allergic neuritis. Ann Neurol 16:680, 1984.
8. Swick HM, McQuillen MP: The use of steroids in the treatment of idiopathic polyneuritis. Neurology 26:205, 1976. (Double blind. Time of onset of illness to recovery was less in steroid-treated patients, although steroids did not change the severity of illness or duration of hospitalization.)
9. Tuck RR, et al: Autonomic dysfunction in Guillain-Barré syndrome. J Neurol Neurosurg Psychiatry 44(11):983, 1981.

PROGRESSIVE DEMENTIA AND MOVEMENT DISORDER

CASE 11: You are asked to see a 45-year-old woman, a 10-year resident of a local psychiatric institution, because of unusual movements. She was initially admitted with depression following a suicide attempt. After treatment of her depression, disorganized behavior and episodic violent outbursts occurred and she was made a ward of the state. For approximately 1 year the staff noted brief, aimless, apparently involuntary movements of her face and limbs, which were unresponsive to a temporary "drug free" holiday (she had been taking chlorpromazine).

Prior to hospitalization, she had intermittently worked as a housekeeper, had lived alone, and had no close friends or known relatives. She had been hospitalized for rheumatic fever at age 12. Medications included thorazine and Elavil.

On examination, she was a frail, withdrawn woman whose speech was limited to single words and who comprehended only one-step commands. There were choreiform movements of the arms, involuntary mouth opening with eyebrow elevation and sudden brief flexions of the neck. Gait was halting and lurching. Power and sensation were normal; reflexes were brisk and plantars were flexor.

NEUROANATOMICAL CLUE:

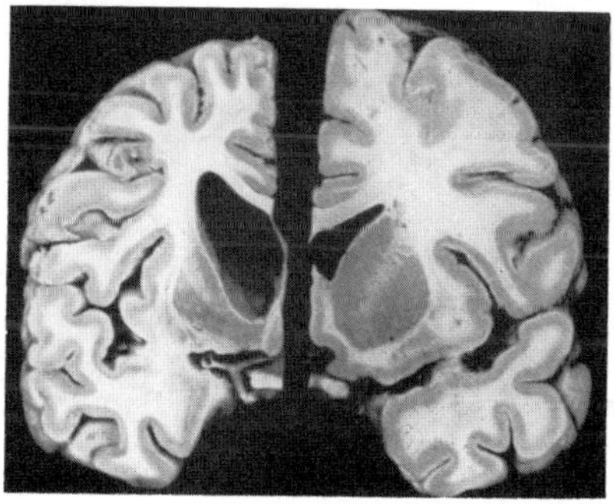

QUESTIONS:

1. What is the possible significance of the history of rheumatic fever in this patient? Why is that unlikely to be the cause of her movement disorder?

2. What involuntary movements are associated with phenothiazines?

3. What is the interpretation of the pathologic findings? What is your diagnosis?

ANSWERS:

1. Acute rheumatic fever may be associated with, or more commonly followed by, Sydenham's chorea. Chorea may follow rheumatic fever by 6 or 12 months but not by 30 years, as in the present case. Furthermore, dementia is not a part of Sydenham's chorea.

2. a) Acute dystonia; b) Parkinsonian-like syndrome (tremor is less common than in idiopathic Parkinson's disease); c) tardive dyskinesia (worm-like movements of tongue, chewing, tongue protrusion, at times associated with involuntary movements of neck, trunk or extremities); d) akathisia (restlessness that may resemble choreoathetosis).

3. Note the profound atrophy of the caudate and putamen on the left brain section (the right brain section is a normal individual shown for comparison)*. These findings are typical of Huntington's chorea. Pathologically, the most prominent finding is a loss of small neurons in the striatum (caudate-putamen).

Capsule - Huntington's Disease (HD)

1. Incidence = 1:100,000

2. Usual onset in fourth to fifth decade, although onset may occur as early as 2 and as late as 71 years of age.

3. Inheritance - Autosomal dominant with nearly complete penetrance.

4. Variants may exist, for example, mental deterioration, seizures and rigidity without chorea (common in childhood HD) or chorea without dementia (late-onset HD).

5. Parents of children at risk for HD may be able to predict which children will develop the disease; impulsivity and emotional instability in childhood may be the forerunner of HD in adulthood.

*(Reproduced with permission from J. H. Adams, J. A. N. Corsellis, and L. W. Duchen: Greenfield's Neuropathology, Edward Arnold Publishers, London, 1963)

6. Neurochemistry of HD - Low levels of GABA in basal ganglia; increased sensitivity to L-dopa.

7. Recently, a gene linked to Huntington's chorea has been identified.

PEARLS:

1. Other rare causes of chorea include hyperthyroidism, birth control pills, and pregnancy.

2. The patient with mild chorea may appear restless and the distinction between restlessness and early chorea can be difficult.

3. Chorea of the tongue can be tested for by asking the patient to maintain the tongue in a protruded position.

4. Hemiballismus - unilateral violent movements - should be distinguished from chorea. Hemiballismus most commonly occurs due to an infarct involving the subthalamic nucleus.

PITFALLS:

1. Suicide is an important cause of death in patients with early HD. Be alert to signs of depression in this population.

2. Polymyoclonus, common with metabolic and some degenerative disorders, is of briefer duration than is chorea, although these two movement disorders may at times be difficult to distinguish from one another.

3. Patients with HD may worsen when given L-dopa. The use of L-dopa as an evocative test in presymptomatic cases of HD should be discouraged.

REFERENCES

1. Chemistry of Huntington's chorea (Editorial). Lancet 1:1119, 1980.
2. Enna SJ, Bird ED, Bennett JP. Huntington's chorea. Changes in neurotransmitter receptors in the brain. N Engl J Med 294:1305, 1976.
3. Gusella JF, Wexler NS, Conneally PM, et al: A polymorphic DNA marker genetically linked to Huntington's disease. Nature 306:234, 1983.
4. Kuhl D, et al: Cerebral metabolism and atrophy in Huntington's disease determined by ^{18}FDG and CT scan. Ann Neurol 12(5):425, 1982.
5. Kurlan R: Clinical impact of recombinant DNA research on neurogenetic diseases. Report of Mary Jennifer Selznick Workshop. Arch Neurol 42:82, 1985.
6. Nausieda PA, et al: Sydenham chorea: An update. Neurology 30:331, 1980.
7. Nemeroff C: Regional brain concentrations of neuropeptides in Huntington's chorea and schizophrenia. Science 221:972, 1983.

BACK PAIN AND LEG WEAKNESS OF ACUTE ONSET

CASE 12: S.K., a 37-year-old married woman previously in good health, had the sudden onset, while walking, of weakness in both legs followed by pain in the midback and chest. The weakness and pain progressed over the next few hours until she could barely move her legs. Her prior history included depression for which she had seen a psychiatrist, but no preceding optic neuritis, transient episodes of paralysis, or numbness.

Her examination included: blood pressure 120/70, pulse 80, temperature 37°C. Her general physical examination was normal except for tenderness over the thoracic spine and a distended bladder. She had normal mentation and cranial nerves, complete paralysis of both lower extremities, normal reflexes in the upper limbs but no reflexes in the lower limbs. There was a sensory level to pin and touch at T5. X-rays of the spine were normal.

NEUROANATOMICAL CLUE:

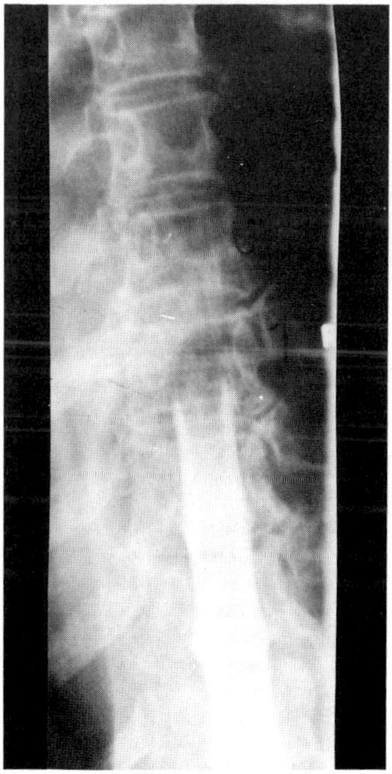

QUESTIONS:

1. What is the differential diagnosis in this case?
2. What does the myelogram show?
3. What are the early symptoms of spinal cord compression?
4. What are the common causes of cord compression?
5. What is the definitive diagnostic test for spinal cord compression?
6. How should this patient be treated?

ANSWERS:

1. Acute spinal cord compression, acute transverse myelopathy, and spinal cord infarction. In transverse myelopathy, the deficit usually evolves slowly (over hours); in patients without a previous history of multiple sclerosis, transverse myelopathy usually is a single event which does not recur. In spinal cord infarction due to occlusion of the anterior spinal artery, there is typically the sudden onset of low thoracic (e.g., T10) motor and sensory deficit sparing posterior column functions of position and vibration sense (supplied by posterior spinal artery).

2. A complete block at T4-5 with failure of the dye column to pass above the level of the block.

3. Local back pain and subtle changes in bladder and bowel function usually precede weakness.

4. Spinal epidural abscess, epidural or subdural hematoma, tumor (usually metastatic), herniated disc.

5. Myelography.

6. Acute cord compression is a surgical emergency; exploration and evacuation of the mass lesion are usually required. The exception to this rule is the case of metastatic tumor from a known primary site; in these cases radiation therapy and high-dose steroids are the initial treatments of choice.

PEARLS:

1. Progressive leg weakness + back pain of sudden onset = spinal cord compression until proven otherwise.

2. Deep tendon reflexes are usually absent in acute cord compression (spinal shock). A sensory level, however, is usually present.

3. Spinal cord compression is an emergency - prognosis is clearly related to the time between onset of symptoms and treatment!

4. Be suspicious of a spinal cord lesion in the patient with cancer who develops back pain, weakness in both legs, or a change in urine or bowel habits.

5. Spinal epidural abscess = back pain, local tenderness and fever; infection may spread to epidural space hematogenously or directly from a contiguous source (e.g., osteomyelitis).

PITFALLS

1. With incomplete spinal cord lesions the sensory "level" on the thorax is often one or two dermatomes below the actual level of the lesion in the spinal cord due to travel of afferent fibers ipsilaterally for several segments after their entry into the cord. Thus, look for spinal cord pathology at least two levels above the "sensory level."

2. Remember, the vertebral body "number" is lower than the corresponding spinal cord segment at that level.

3. All patients with distended bladder from acute spinal cord disease will require catheterization.

4. In early spinal cord compression, local pain may be the only presenting symptom. A psychiatric (functional) origin for acute neurologic symptoms should be considered only after organic possibilities have been excluded. (In the above case, a psychiatric etiology was the initial consideration.)

REFERENCES

1. Baker AS, Ojemann RG, Swartz MN, Richardson EP Jr. Spinal epidural abscess. N Engl J Med 293:463, 1975.
2. Gilbert RW, Kim J-H, Posner JB. Epidural spinal cord compression from metastatic tumor: diagnosis and treatment. Ann Neurol 3:40, 1978.
3. Foo D, Rossier AB: Preoperative neurological status in predicting surgical outcome of spinal subdural hematomas. Surg Neurol 15:389, 1981.
4. Rodriguez M, Dinapoli R: Epidural cord compression with special reference to metastatic epidural tumors. Mayo Clin Proc 55:442, 1980.
5. Roscoe MW: Acute spinal subdural hematoma: a case report and review of the literature. Spine 9:672, 1984.

CLUMSINESS, VISUAL LOSS, AND PARESTHESIAS IN A YOUNG MAN

CASE 13: A 24-year-old graduate student came to his physician because of difficulty walking of three months' duration. In addition to having a clumsy gait, the patient reported an episode of "heaviness" and "tingling" in his right arm that had occurred three years previously. When he was 18 years old, he had temporarily lost vision in his right eye. Abnormalities on neurologic exam included slurring of speech, pallor of the right optic disc, "finger-to-nose" ataxia of the right upper extremity, and exaggerated reflexes at the knees and ankles with extensor plantar responses. Reflexes were normoactive in the upper extremities, and sensory exam was normal.

NEUROANATOMICAL CLUE:

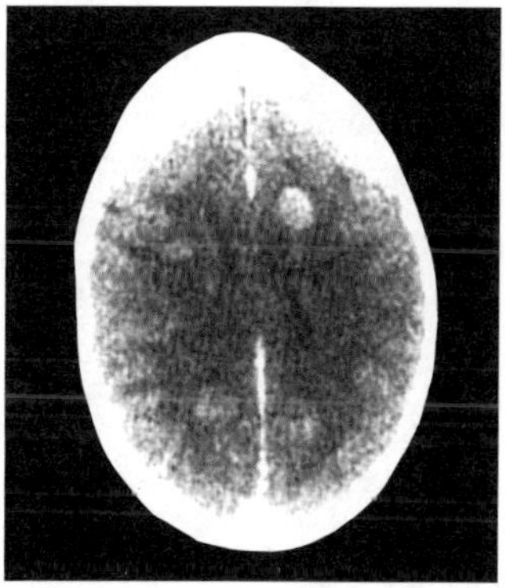

QUESTIONS:

1. What is the most likely diagnosis? What are the two major clinical forms of this disease?

2. What are typical abnormalities of cerebrospinal fluid in this condition? What other laboratory features might be helpful in establishing the diagnosis?

3. What is the presumed etiology of this disease?

4. What is the prognosis?

5. What is the treatment of choice?

ANSWERS:

1. Multiple sclerosis (MS). Major clinical forms: relapsing-remitting disease and chronic-progressive disease.

2. Elevated CSF gamma globulin and oligoclonal immunoglobulin bands are characteristic. A low-grade mononuclear pleocytosis (5-20 cells/mm^3) may be present when disease is active. A CT scan with contrast may show the presence of multiple enhancing white matter lesions. The CT scan on this patient showed a periventricular plaque adjacent to the right frontal horn, 2 plaques posteriorly, and the suggestion of a plaque adjacent to the left ventricle. Magnetic resonance imaging is the most sensitive radiographic test to demonstrate MS plaques. Evoked responses (visual, auditory and somatosensory) often demonstrate delays in conduction in these pathways.

3. An autoimmune attack against central nervous system white matter, probably related to an antecedent viral infection.

4. Prognosis is uncertain; approximately one-third of patients can expect to lead full, normal lives with little incapacity; another third have severe disease with complete disability, the other third a course intermediate between these two groups. The clinical course during the first 5 years after diagnosis is often a good indicator of the long-range prognosis.

5. Steroids (ACTH or corticosteroids) are given during acute attacks. ACTH appears to speed the rate of recovery from acute MS attacks, although neither ACTH or corticosteroid therapy has been shown to change the long-term prognosis. Most experimental therapies involve some form of immunosuppression. Chronic progressive disease is the most disabling form and may be temporarily halted in some patients by a short course of high-dose cyclophosphamide.

PEARLS:

1. An internuclear ophthalmoplegia (INO), due to a lesion of the medial longitudinal fasciculus (which connects the sixth and third cranial nerve nuclei), is a hallmark of the disease. An INO consists of a delay in movement of the AD-ducting eye and nystagmus in the AB-ducting eye. Remember, an INO indicates a periventricular lesion at the upper pons - midbrain level IPSILATERALLY. Bilateral INO is almost pathognomonic of MS; unilateral INO may be due to vascular disease or tumor.

2. Check for the presence of an increased jaw jerk in patients with hyperreflexia; if present, there is a lesion above the midpons.

3. Brief (seconds - minutes) paroxysms of numbness, weakness, spasms or involuntary movements are common in MS patients and may respond to carbamazepine.

4. Heat typically makes MS patients neurologically worse and cold exposure may improve function. A "hot bath" was formerly used as a provocative test for MS.

5. One-third to two-thirds of patients who present with isolated optic neuritis will subsequently develop multiple sclerosis.

6. Fatigue is a very common symptom in patients with MS and may be helped by amantadine, 100 mg twice a day.

PITFALLS:

1. Rule out disc disease and spinal cord tumor in all patients with progressive myelopathy.

2. Lhermitte's sign consists of electric shock-like sensations down the back and into legs evoked by neck flexion. Although common in MS, it may also be present in other conditions, such as cervical disc disease.

3. "Tic doloureux" in a young patient may be due to multiple sclerosis, particularly if the pain is atypical or bilateral.

4. Depression in the MS patient may present with vague complaints of increased weakness and fatigue; these symptoms often respond to appropriate therapy.

REFERENCES

1. Barrett L, Drayer B, Shin C: High resolution computed tomography in multiple sclerosis. Ann Neurol 17:33, 1985.
2. Ellison GW, Wisscher BR, Graves MC, Fahey JL: UCLA Conference on Multiple Sclerosis. Ann Intern Med 101:514, 1984.
3. Hauser SL, Dawson DM, Lehrich JR, Beal MF, Kevy SV, Propper RD, Mills JA, Weiner HL: Intensive immunosuppression in progressive multiple sclerosis. A randomized, three-arm study of high-dose intravenous cyclophosphamide, plasma exchange, and ACTH. N Engl J Med 308:173, 1983.
4. McAlpine D, Lumsden CE, Acheson ED. Multiple Sclerosis: A Reappraisal. Edinburgh, ES Livingstone Ltd., 1965.
5. McFarlin DE, McFarland HF: Multiple sclerosis. N Engl J Med 307:1183-1188, 1246-1251, 1982.
6. Weiner HL, Hauser SL: Neuroimmunology I: Immunoregulation in neurological disease. Ann Neurol 11:437, 1982.

HEADACHE, OBESITY, AND BLINDNESS

CASE 14: You are asked to see a 26-year-old woman with persistent headaches and bilateral visual loss. Several years ago she developed intermittent headaches relieved by rest. One year ago she became unable to see clearly out of the right eye; this was followed by progressive worsening of vision in that eye. Three months ago she noted difficulty with reading in the left eye, and she is now unable to read at all. For the past year, she has been amenorrheic. She has been obese since age 12, and over the past 5 years has gained 50 pounds. She took birth control pills for a 6-month period 5 years ago, but stopped because of headache. On examination, pupils were 5 mm and slightly reactive, vision was restricted to small islands of preserved light perception in the superior visual fields, and there was bilateral optic atrophy. Remainder of the neurologic exam was normal.

NEUROANATOMICAL CLUE:

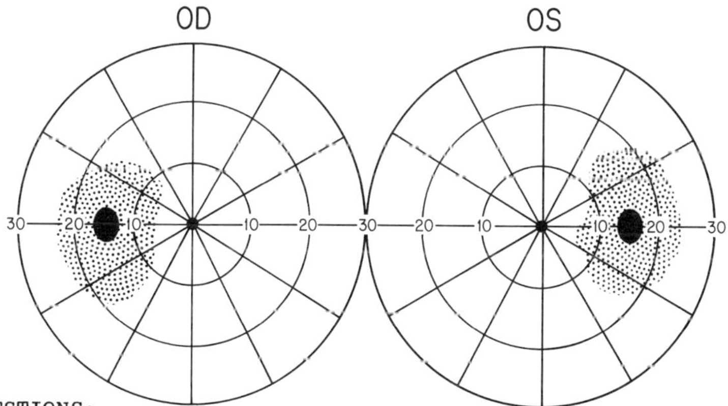

QUESTIONS:

1. How does the CT scan help narrow the diagnosis?

2. You next perform a lumbar puncture. Results: opening pressure 350 mm Hg; acellular; protein 15 mg%, sugar 80 mg%. What is your diagnosis?

3. What are other important causes of progressive visual loss in young adults?

4. What is the presumed etiology of her disorder?

5. What is the treatment?

ANSWERS:

1. A <u>normal CT scan</u> rules out a mass lesion or hydrocephalus.

2. <u>Benign intracranial hypertension</u> (pseudotumor cerebri).

3. Think of: a) <u>compressive</u> lesions - pituitary adenoma (bitemporal hemianopsia), meningioma, neurofibroma; b) <u>inflammatory</u> lesions such as multiple sclerosis (usually attacks of visual loss rather than slowly progressive loss), or chronic basilar meningitis; c) <u>familial</u> etiology - Leber's optic atrophy.

4. Brain edema; i.e., an increase in brain volume secondary to increased water content. CSF absorption may be impaired.

5. Treatment depends upon the severity of the illness (e.g., is there visual loss?) and the underlying cause (if known). Weight loss, periodic lumbar punctures, drugs to reduce CSF production (acetazolamide, furosamide), and steroids would be reasonable measures in this patient. If these treatments fail to reduce intracranial pressure, surgical decompression is indicated.

PEARLS:

1. <u>Enlarged blind spots</u> are seen on visual field examination and sudden obscurations of vision, lasting up to 15 seconds, are common. Neuroanatomical clue illustrates enlarged blind spots.

2. <u>Headache</u> is usually but not always present. Headache is typically worse in the early morning, may be accentuated by cough but is <u>not</u> associated with vomiting or meningismus.

3. <u>Mental status</u> is normal in benign intracranial hypertension. Examination reveals no localizing findings. Non-localizing findings, including visual loss or 6th cranial nerve palsy, may be present.

4. Benign intracranial hypertension is 5-10 times <u>more common in women</u> than in men and is rare after age 50.

5. Benign intracranial hypertension may be a cause of the <u>empty sella syndrome</u>.

6. CSF protein is often below normal in benign intracranial hypertension.

PITFALLS:

1. Do not miss treatable conditions which may be associated with the development of benign intracranial hypertension:

   a) Endocrine - Obesity, menstrual irregularities, birth control pills, Addison's disease, hypoparathyroidism, steroid withdrawal.

   b) Drugs - Vitamin A, tetracycline, nalidixic acid.

   c) Venous sinus thrombosis - Associated with mastoiditis, head trauma, pregnancy.

   d) Blood disorders - Iron deficiency anemia.

2. Note: A common result in the workup of a "pseudotumor" suspect is discovery of a tumor.

REFERENCES

1. Ahlskog JE, O'Neill BP: Pseudotumor cerebri. Ann Int Med 97:249, 1982.
2. Boddie HG, Banna M, Bradley WG: "Benign" intracranial hypertension. A survey of the clinical and radiological features, and long-term prognosis. Brain 97:313, 1974.
3. Fishman RA: Cerebrospinal Fluid in Diseases of the Nervous System. Philadelphia, W.B. Saunders, 1980.
4. Johnston I, Paterson A: Benign intracranial hypertension. I. Diagnosis and prognosis. Brain 97:289, 1974.
5. Rush JA: Pseudotumor cerebri: clinical profile and visual outcome in 63 patients. Mayo Clin Proc 55:541, 1980.
6. Spector RH, Carlisle J: Pseudotumor cerebri caused by a synthetic vitamin A preparation. Neurology 34:1509, 1984.
7. Weisberg LA: Benign intracranial hypertension. Medicine 54:197, 1975.

FEVER AND OBTUNDATION

<u>CASE 15</u>: A 21-year-old woman was a known drug dealer and intravenous drug abuser. She was brought to the emergency room after being found on the floor of her apartment by friends. Examination revealed an obtunded, febrile (39.6) woman; there were two nailbed splinter hemorrhages, a grade II systolic ejection murmur, and a palpable spleen tip. The patient did not respond to commands and was in a sleep-like state; eyes were tonically deviated to the left. She would open her eyes when pinched and push away the examiner. Both optic discs were blurred and raised, there was a right hemianopsia to threat and a right hemiparesis involving face, arm, and leg.

NEUROANATOMICAL CLUE:

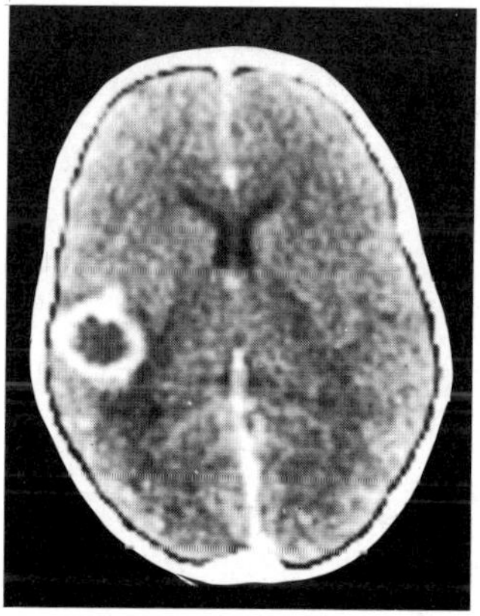

QUESTIONS:

1. What is the significance of enhancement on the CAT scan?
2. What is the most likely diagnosis?
3. List several causes of this condition.
4. What is the appropriate treatment?

ANSWERS:

1. Enhancing lesions on CT scan = abnormalities of the blood-brain barrier. Think of tumor, inflammation (infection), or arteriovenous malformation.

2. Brain abscess. Fever, cardiac murmur, palpable spleen tip and splinter hemmorhages suggest bacterial endocarditis, a common complication of intravenous drug abuse. In this patient, brain abscess was likely due to hematogenous spread of infection from an infected heart valve.

3. Pathogenesis of brain abscess:

Origin		Location of Abscess
A. Contiguous spread (40%):		
Frontal sinus	to	Frontal lobe
Maxillary sinus	to	Temporal lobe
Ethmoid sinus	to	Cerebellum or temporal lobe
B. Hematogenous (35%):		
From lungs (lung abscess, emphysema), Heart (infected valve or right to left shunt), or other infected site		May be multiple; frequently distal middle cerebral artery distribution
C. Direct inoculation:		
Following open brain trauma or surgery (5%)		Abscess corresponds to site of injury
D. Idiopathic		

4. The organisms most common in brain abscesses are anaerobic streptococci and bacteroids. A commonly used therapeutic regimen consists of penicillin (20 x 10^6 units/day) and chloramphenicol (4-6 gr daily). If penicillinase-producing staphylococci are suspected, a semi-synthetic penicillin (e.g., nafcillin) is usually added. Traditionally, surgical drainage of abscess cavities was routinely performed, but many centers now reserve surgery for cases in which: a) the diagnosis is uncertain; b) the abscess is very large or associated with persistent raised

intracranial pressure; or c) there is a poor response to medical therapy. Serial CT scans can help assess the response of brain abscesses to medical therapy.

PEARLS:

1. Headache, focal neurologic signs, and expanding intracranial lesions - think of brain abscess.

2. In patients with acute or severe brain injury:

   - Eye deviation away from hemiparesis = cerebral hemisphere injury.

   - Eye deviation towards hemiparesis = brainstem injury.

PITFALLS:

1. In established brain abscess, <u>temperature and white blood count may be normal</u>.

2. When faced with <u>sudden deterioration</u> in patients with brain abscess, think of: a) herniation, or b) rupture into a ventricle.

3. When raised intracranial pressure is suspected, a CT scan should precede lumbar puncture. The exception to this rule is when there is a strong possbility of bacterial meningitis. In patients with suspected brain abscess, lumbar puncture is extremely dangerous.

REFERENCES

1. Bell WE: Treatment of bacterial infection of the central nervous system. Ann Neurol 9:313, 1981.
2. Rosenblum ML, Hoff JT, Norman D, Weinstein PR, Pitts L: Decreased mortality of brain abscess since advent of computerized tomography. J Neurosurg 49:658, 1978.
3. Yang S-Y: Brain abscess: a review of 400 cases. J Neurosurg 55:794, 1981.
4. Weissberg LA: Nonsurgical management of focal intracranial infection. Neurology 31:575, 1981.

HEADACHE AND LEFT HEMIPARESIS

CASE 16: A 59-year-old man was well until 2 months prior to admission, when he developed early morning headaches which would awaken him from sleep. Although the headaches typically disappeared shortly after arising from bed, the severity of the headaches was increasing with time. Two days earlier he developed progressive weakness of his left hand and an unstable gait. Past medical history was notable for a malignant melanoma which was discovered on his right arm 2 years previously and treated with local resection and a radical axillary lymph node dissection. Review of systems revealed weight loss of 15 pounds over the past month.

On examination, the patient was alert, although confused and unable to give a coherent history. Fundoscopic examination revealed bilateral papilledema. There was nearly complete paralysis of the left arm and mild weakness of the proximal left leg. There was a left facial asymmetry. Reflexes were increased on the left and plantar responses were extensor bilaterally. Sensory examination was normal. The remainder of the cranial nerves were normal. Gait was stable, although the patient had a tendency to fall when turning rapidly. A CT scan was performed.

NEUROANATOMICAL CLUE:

QUESTIONS:

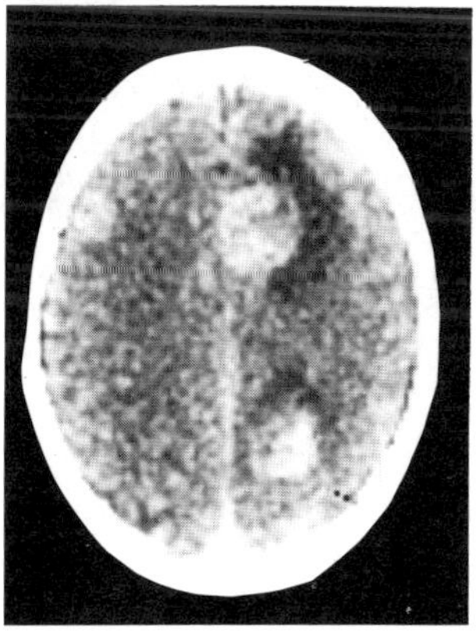

1. What is the most likely cause of this patient's symptoms?
2. What is the significance of his headache?
3. What is the significance of papilledema?
4. What further investigations are indicated?
5. What is the appropriate treatment?
6. What is the prognosis?

ANSWERS:

1. The CT scan shows multiple areas of increased density in both hemispheres. The largest abnormality is seen in the right frontal lobe and is surrounded by an area of edema; other lesions are seen in the right parietal and temporal and left frontal regions. This is the CT picture of metastatic tumor.

2. Early morning headache which improves on rising is characteristic of raised intracranial pressure.

3. Papilledema or swelling of the optic disc is an important sign of raised intracranial pressure. In mild form, papilledema can be detected by an absence of the venous pulsations in the disc and by a blurring and elevation of the disc margin. In more advanced forms, swelling of the entire disc with venous congestion and peripapillary hemorrhages are found. Papilledema secondary to raised intracranial pressure is usually bilateral. Patients with papilledema generally have normal or nearly normal vision with an enlarged blind spot and constriction of the visual fields; preserved visual acuity is an important distinguishing feature between papilledema and papillitis (optic neuritis). In optic neuritis, visual acuity is usually severely impaired.

4. Cerebral metastases usually occur in the setting of widely disseminated cancer; thus, investigations to determine the extent of cancer spread are indicated. In addition, biopsy of an accessible lesion is indicated for confirmation of the diagnosis. In this patient, chest X-ray revealed metastatic lesions in lung and bone, and a rib biopsy revealed metastatic malignant melanoma.

5. Multiple brain metastases are treated with steroids (e.g., dexamethasone 10 mg IV bolus followed by 4 mg po q6h) and radiation therapy. The majority of treated patients experience a stabilization or improvement of their neurologic condition following treatment. In patients with a single brain metastasis and little or medically treatable systemic disease, surgical resection combined with radiotherapy may be effective.

6. The prognosis is poor. The median life expectancy is 12 weeks for patients with brain metastases; the prognosis may be somewhat better for patients with breast cancer. The majority of patients with brain metastasis die of complications from systemic cancer rather than from the direct effects of the brain tumor.

PEARLS:

1. Neuropathy of the mental nerve ("numb chin syndrome") in the absence of trauma is usually due to metastatic cancer to the mandible. It may be the presenting symptom in the patient with cancer.

2. Brain metastases which have a tendency to bleed include choriocarcinoma, melanoma, bronchogenic carcinoma, and renal cell carcinoma.

3. Metastatic cancer to the meninges (carcinomatous meningitis) typically produces headache, backache, confusion, radicular pain, and cranial nerve palsies. Meningeal tumor implants may be visualized by CT scan and malignant cells may be recovered in the cerebrospinal fluid.

4. Brain metastases generally develop from hematogenous spread of tumor. Metastases to the skull may develop from spread via Batson's plexus, a series of veins which run the length of the vertebral column to the venous sinuses of the skull.

5. The most common presenting symptoms of brain metastases are: headache, motor weakness, mental changes, ataxia, and seizures.

PITFALLS:

1. Rapid neurological deterioration in the patient with suspected brain metastasis can occur and should be treated with osmotic agents (mannitol), steroids (dexamethasone 10 mg IV bolus, then 4 mg qid), and hyperventilation.

2. Beware of the fact that in a patient with a known primary systemic tumor and a brain lesion that the latter may be a separate process (e.g., meningioma, subdural, brain abscess).

REFERENCES

1. Cairncross JG, Kim J-H, Posner JB: Radiation therapy for brain metastases. Ann Neurol 7:529, 1980.
2. Castaldo JE, et al: Intracranial metastases due to prostatic carcinoma. Cancer 51:1739, 1983.
3. Greenberg HS: Metastases to the base of the skull: Clinical findings in 43 patients. Neurology 31:530, 1981.
4. Jaeckle KA, Krol G, Posner JB: Evaluation of computed tomographic abnormalities in leptomeningeal metastases. Ann Neurol 17:85, 1985.
5. Mandybur TI: Intracranial hemorrhage caused by metastatic tumors. Neurology 27:650, 1977.
6. Massey EW, Moore J, Schold SC Jr: Mental neuropathy from systemic cancer. Neurology 31:1277, 1981.

TREMOR

CASE 17:

A) A 67-year-old retired government employee was brought by his wife because of "shaking." The wife reported that not only did his hands shake, but there had been a recent personality change. The patient had become very "slow" in his movements and often sat motionless with an expressionless face. Examination showed a 3 per second resting tremor that improved with movement. There was cogwheel rigidity of the limbs and a shuffling gait. The patient was alert and intelligent and the remainder of the examination was normal.

B) A 53 year old furniture salesman came to his doctor because of a tremor involving his upper extremities. He had had the tremor for over 20 years but it was not disabling. He sought medical advice because his son was beginning to develop a similar tremor. The father's tremor was most pronounced when he became excited or tried to write something important. Once he found himself unable to write a check. The tremor improved whenever he drank alcohol. Examination showed the tremor to be worse when his arms were extended, better at rest. In addition, there was a mild tremor of the head. Neurologic examination was otherwise normal.

QUESTIONS:

1. What is the diagnosis in case A? What are the cardinal features of that disease?

2. What is the diagnosis in case B? What is the most effective treatment?

3. What is the differential diagnosis of action tremor?

4. What are the important drugs used to treat Parkinson's disease? What is the "neuropharmacologic" abnormality?

5. What is tardive dyskinesia? What is the best treatment?

ANSWERS:

1. Parkinson's disease. Tremor, rigidity, and bradykinesia.

2. Action tremor (familial tremor). Propranolol is the drug of choice.

3. Hyperthyroidism, pheochromocytoma, and stimulant drugs (amphetamines, caffeine) may also produce action tremor. This type of tremor is due to alternate contractions and relaxations in agonist and antagonist muscle groups and in this respect is identical to physiologic (e.g., normal) tremor and to the tremor which appears with normal fatigue.

4. L-dopa, generally given with carbidopa, a peripheral dopa decarboxylase inhibitor (Sinemet), is the most important drug in the treatment of patients with Parkinson's disease. Other medications include anticholinergics (Artane, Cogentin), amantadine and bromocriptine. In general, the initial drug of choice for the patient with mild Parkinson's disease is Sinemet or anticholinergic medication. Many clinicians prefer to delay L-dopa therapy until the patient has functional/psychological problems not controlled with less potent anti-parkinsonian agents. For patients with moderate to severe symptoms, Sinemet is the drug of choice and anticholinergics, amantadine, and bromocriptine are ancillary drugs for patients whose symptoms are poorly controlled with Sinemet alone or for patients who experience toxicity from Sinemet therapy. The key neuropharmacologic abnormality in Parkinson's disease is decreased dopaminergic activity in the brain, especially involving the substantia nigra and its projections to the basal ganglia. Therefore, treatment corrects this abnormality by increasing dopaminergic activity (Sinemet, amantadine, bromocriptine) or, conversely, by decreasing cholinergic activity.

5. Tardive dyskinesia usually consists of involuntary movements of the face and mouth and may also involve neck, trunk, and extremities. Tardive dyskinesia is a complication of chronic neuropleptic drug use (e.g., phenothiazines) and may be associated with acute dystonias or parkinsonian-like syndromes in these patients. There is no consistently effective treatment for most patients with tardive dyskinesias,

although withdrawal of the offending drug is the most logical treatment for most patients. Depletion of brain dopamine (e.g., by drugs like reserpine) may be useful. Tardive dyskinesia may also be seen in elderly patients without preceding phenothiazine use.

PEARLS:

1. Frequent small doses of L-dopa may be needed for successful treatment of Parkinson's disease.

2. Neurologic examination is otherwise normal in patients with action tremor.

3. Action tremor improves with alcohol.

4. Other important symptoms of Parkinson's disease include a shuffling gait, drooling, and softening of voice to a whisper or mumbling. Lack of arm swing and infrequency of blinking (normally 15-20 times per minute) may be early signs.

5. The tremor of Parkinson's disease is slow (3-6 per second) and the tremor improves with movement and is worse at rest.

6. Progressive dementia may be associated with moderate to severe Parkinson's disease.

7. The pathology of Parkinson's disease - loss of pigmented cells in the central nervous system (substantia nigra, locus ceruleus, motor portion of the vagus nerve). Cytoplasmic inclusions (Lewy bodies) may be present in remaining cells.

8. A severe, rapidly-evolving parkinsonian syndrome has recently been described in individuals manufacturing or using illicit narcotics, and the toxic metabolite responsible for this syndrome has now been identified.

PITFALLS:

1. Remember that slow and infrequent movement may be a sign of depression (not all patients with hypokinesia have extrapyramidal disease).

2. The abrupt stopping of anticholinergic therapy can lead to dramatic deterioration in patients with Parkinson's disease.

3. Side effects of L-dopa therapy include the development of involuntary movements and sudden dramatic worsening of parkinsonian symptoms (on-off effect). Patients with these side effects may benefit from lower doses given more frequently or periodic drug-free "holidays."

4. Patients with extrapyramidal symptoms and eye movement abnormalities (in particular a loss of voluntary downgaze) may be suffering from a related degenerative disorder, progressive supernuclear palsy.

REFERENCES

1. Boshes B: Sinemet and the treatment of Parkinsonism. Ann Intern Med 94:364, 1981.
2. Burns RS, Chiueh CC, Markey SP, Ebert MH, Jacobowity DM, Kopin IJ: A primate model of Parkinsonism: selective destruction of dopaminergic neurons in the pars compacta of the substantia nigra by N-methyl-4-phenyl-1,2,3,6-tetrahydropyridine. Proc Natl Acad Sci USA 80:4546, 1984.
3. Fahn S (Ed): Management of Parkinson's Disease at Different Stages of the Illness. Clin Neuropharmacol 5(Suppl 1), 1982.
4. Hoehn MM: Low dosage of bromocriptine added to Levodopa in Parkinson's disease. Neurology 35:199, 1985.
5. Lieberman A, et al: Dementia in Parkinson's disease. Ann Neurol 6:355, 1979.
6. Nutt JG, Woodward WR, Hammerstad JP, Carter JH, Anderson JL: The "on-off" phenomenon in Parkinson's disease: relation to Levodopa absorption and transport. N Engl J Med 310:483, 1984.
7. Rajput AH, Stern W, Laverty WH: Chronic low-dose Levodopa therapy in Parkinson's disease: An argument for delaying Levodopa therapy. Neurology 34:991, 1984.
8. Weiner WJ, Koller WC, Peruk S, Nausieda PA, Klawans HL: Drug holiday and management of Parkinson's disease. Neurology 30:1257, 1980.

ABDOMINAL PAIN AND LOSS OF CONSCIOUSNESS

CASE 18: A 70-year-old woman had the sudden onset of nausea and abdominal pain. She then lost consciousness and became incontinent. She awakened 5 minutes later, but was lethargic and confused. Further questioning revealed that she had fallen and struck her head 6 weeks earlier and had fractured four ribs. General examination was normal and there were no focal findings on neurological exam. Routine CBC and blood studies were normal. Skull X-ray, CT scan, and lumbar puncture were normal. An EEG was performed and is shown below.

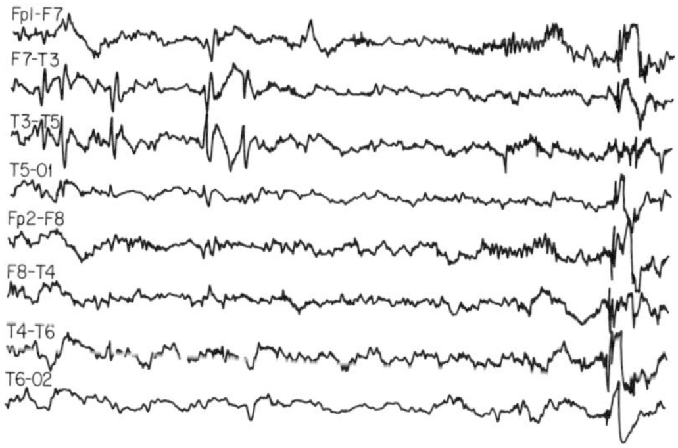

QUESTIONS:

1. What is the cause of the patient's abdominal pain and loss of consciousness?
2. When do post-traumatic seizures usually occur?
3. What are some metabolic causes of seizures?
4. Give examples of the auras associated with partial complex (temporal lobe) epilepsy.
5. Which are the major drugs for focal seizures? For petit mal?
6. For how long should anticonvulsants be continued?

ANSWERS:

1. Posttraumatic temporal lobe seizure with visceral aura.

2. Most posttraumatic seizures develop during the first year after injury. The risk of developing post-traumatic seizures is proportional to the extent of brain injury; approximately 40-50% of patients with dural penetration or with unconsciousness of greater than 24 hours will develop post-traumatic seizures, whereas patients with closed head injuries and those without significant amnesia have a lower incidence of subsequent seizures.

3. Think of the three "HYPOS" - hypoglycemia, hypocalcemia, and hyponatremia, as well as renal and hepatic disease.

4. Dizziness, vertigo, nausea, unpleasant odors, deja vu, jamais vu, micropsia (objects shrinking), macropsia (objects enlarging), the sensation of time speeding up, formed sensory hallucinations (auditory or visual), emotions (fear, anger), a sense of depersonalization, forced thinking or paranoid ideation, specific memories, automatisms (for example, lip smacking, aimless walking, picking at clothes) and the unconscious performance of skilled activities such as driving a car.

5. Diphenylhydantoin (Dilantin), carbamazepine (Tegretol), primidone (Mysoline). Petit mal is treated with ethosuximide or valproic acid (Depakene).

6. Anticonvulsants may be discontinued in patients who have been seizure-free for at least 4 years, who have normal neurological examinations, and whose EEGs have no paroxysmal discharges.

PEARLS:

1. Clue shows a spike focus in the temporal lobe. Remember, there are two types of seizures - focal (partial) and generalized. Most seizures that begin in adulthood are focal seizures. Focal seizures imply that there is an abnormality in the electrical activity of a localized portion of cerebral cortex; the development of a focal seizure disorder should

initiate a search for local pathology. Generalized seizures have no focal components, usually begin in childhood, and include petit mal and idiopathic grand mal epilepsy.

2. The best historian in a seizure workup is a witness, not the patient.

3. Trauma is a major cause of acquired epilepsy.

4. Anticonvulsant drug levels are important in the effective treatment of patients with seizure disorders. The availability of anticonvulsant blood levels has improved the control of seizures by at least 50%. They should be drawn if seizure frequency suddenly increases, if signs of possible drug toxicity appear, or when patient compliance is questionable.

5. Patients with seizures need considerable emotional and social support. Personality disorders are associated with temporal lobe epilepsy and may require psychotropic drugs.

6. A seizure discharge is due to the synchronous firing of neurons in a localized area of brain. Under normal circumstances gamma-aminobutyric acid (GABA) is thought to be an inhibitory neurotransmitter in the brain; many anticonvulsants are believed to act by enhancing GABA inhibition.

PITFALLS:

1. In patients who experience exacerbations of a seizure disorder, think of: a) failure to take medications, b) infection, c) subdural hematoma, d) alcohol.

2. Simplify anticonvulsant regimens as much as possible. Do not add additional anticonvulsants unless the anticonvulsant(s) that the patient is already taking is (are) in therapeutic range (check blood levels).

3. A temporal lobe seizure can be the first manifestation of acute herpes simplex encephalitis or of a brain tumor.

4. Be aware of the complications of commonly used anticonvulsants. For example, agranulocytosis is a rare complication of carbamazepine, and periodic blood counts are important in patients receiving this drug.

5. It is the physician's responsibility to advise patients with recent seizures to check with their state motor vehicle bureau regarding the local laws concerning driving. In most states, patients are not permitted to drive within 1 year of a generalized seizure.

REFERENCES

1. Bridgers SL, Ebersole JS: The clinical utility of ambulatory cassette EEG monitoring. Neurology 35:166, 1985.
2. Delgado-Escuta AV, Treiman DM, Walsh GO: The treatable epilepsies. N Engl J Med 308:1508 (Part I); 308:1576 (Part II), 1983.
3. Dichter MA: The epilepsies and convulsive disorders. In Principles of Internal Medicine, Petersdorf, et al (Eds), 10th edition, New York, McGraw-Hill, 1983.
4. Goldenshones (Ed): Changing Approaches to the Management of Seizures: Pharmacologic Considerations. Epilepsia 23(Suppl 1), 1982.
5. So EL, Penry JK: Epilepsy in adults. Ann Neurol 9:3, 1981.
6. Solomon G, Plum F: Clinical Management of Seizures. A Guide for the Physician. Saunders, Philadephia, 1983.
7. Thurston JH, Thurston DL, Hixon BB, Keller AJ: Prognosis in childhood epilepsy. Additional follow-up of 148 children 15-23 years after withdrawal of anticonvulsant therapy. N Engl J Med 306:831, 1982.

SEIZURES AND CONFUSION

CASE 19:

A) A 46-year-old businessman was brought to the emergency room because of a seizure. Friends reported that he had been drinking heavily for 6 months, but 2 days earlier told them that he was "going to quit." A witness said that his seizure began as a generalized convulsion involving both arms and legs; the seizure lasted 3-5 minutes. In the emergency room, he was sleepy but arousable; general physical and neurologic examination was normal. In the next half hour the patient awoke. The examination remained within normal limits.

B) You are asked to see a 57-year-old woman with confusion. She is a chronic alcoholic and has been hospitalized multiple times previously. On this occasion, she was admitted one day earlier because of pneumonia and dehydration. She was treated overnight with hydration and antibiotics. The nurses noted the following morning that she had become markedly confused. On examination she was a very thin, apparently malnourished woman who was lethargic and apathetic and would frequently fall off to sleep when questioned. She was disoriented to time and place and gave irrational answers to simple questions. There was a prominent vertical and horizontal nystagmus and a left sixth cranial nerve palsy. The optic discs were within normal limits. Her gait was broad based and ankle jerks were absent. The remainder of the neurologic examination was within normal limits.

QUESTIONS:

1. What is the most likely cause of the seizure in the 46-year-old businessman?

2. What is the appropriate therapy?

3. How would you treat the 57-year-old woman?

4. What is the probable relationship between the medical therapy administered to the woman and her acute neurological illness?

5. Why were the ankle reflexes absent in both patients?

ANSWERS:

1. Alcohol withdrawal seizures or "rum fits." These are generally brief and self-limited seizures that occur 12-48 hours following the cessation of drinking; they are generally preceded by tremulousness.

2. No specific therapy is necessary for uncomplicated alcohol withdrawal seizures. Supportive measures, including adequate hydration and monitoring electrolytes (including serum calcium and magnesium), are indicated. If seizures persist, however, anticonvulsants should be administered and a search for other causes for the seizures initiated (e.g., head trauma).

3. This patient has acute Wernicke's disease, which consists of nystagmus and other oculomotor abnormalities, gait ataxia, and confusional state. This thiamine-deficiency syndrome responds to thiamine (50 mg i.v. and 50 mg i.m. initial dose). Wernicke's disease may coexist with delirium tremens.

4. The administration of intravenous glucose can precipitate Wernicke's disease in alcoholics; all at-risk patients should receive thiamine prior to glucose.

5. Absent ankle reflexes signify a peripheral neuropathy which, in these patients, is due to the combined effects of alcohol and malnutrition. Alcoholic neuropathy is usually asymptomatic but may produce painful burning feet. The treatment of alcoholic polyneuropathy consists of abstinence from alcohol, a balanced diet, and vitamin supplementation. Check B_{12} level.

PEARLS:

1. The most serious complication of alcohol withdrawal is delirium tremens (DTs), which consist of tremulousness, disorientation with hallucinations, perspiration, and autonomic hyperactivity. DTs generally begin 3-5 days after cessation of drinking. Rum fits may herald DTs, but seizures are not a usual manifestation of DTs.

2. Hallucinations accompanying alcoholic withdrawal tend to be visual and frequently involve hallucinations of small animals (microzooanotic

hallucinosis). In Wernicke's encephalopathy the ocular abnormalities resolve within hours following therapy.

3. Korsakoff's psychosis is a further complication of untreated thiamine deficiency in alcoholics and usually includes chronic amnesia and confabulation.

4. Other complications of alcoholism include: cerebellar degeneration, proximal myopathy, central pontine myelinolysis, and demyelination of the corpus collosum (Marchiafava-Bignami).

5. In several large autopsy series of the general population the incidence of Wernicke's disease was 2%, a much higher incidence than recognized during life. Think of Wernicke's disease in all alcoholic and malnourished patients.

PITFALLS:

1. Alcohol withdrawal seizures are nonfocal. If an alcoholic has a focal seizure, it implies underlying pathology, whether a scar from previous head trauma, a brain tumor, or subdural hematoma.

2. In alcoholics who develop new neurological symptoms, think of: a) subdural hematoma; b) infection (pneumonia, meningitis); c) metabolic derangements (thiamine deficiency, hypoglycemia).

3. Patients who die in acute delirium tremens generally have a complicating illness (subdural hematoma, infection), or have severe electrolyte imbalance.

REFERENCES

1. Behse F, Buchtal F: Alcoholic neuropathy: clinical, electrophysiological and biopsy findings. Ann Neurol 2:95, 1977.
2. Endo Y, Oda M, Hara M: Central pontine myelinosis. A study of 37 cases in 1,000 consecutive autopsies. Acta Neuropath (Berl.) 53:145, 1981.
3. Koeppen AG, Barren KD: Marchiofava-Bignami disease. Neurology 28:290, 1978.
4. Nakada T, Knight RT: Alcohol and the central nervous system. Med Clin North Am 68:121, 1984.
5. Thompson WL: Management of alcohol withdrawal syndromes. Arch Int Med 138:278, 1978.
6. Victor M, Adams RD, Collins G: *The Wernicke-Korsakoff Syndrome*, Philadelphia, F.A. Davis, 1971.

DIPLOPIA AND INCONTINENCE

CASE 20:

A) A 53-year-old businessman with no previous medical history suddenly complained of pain over his right eye and "saw double" one afternoon while at work. The double vision disappeared when he covered his right eye. Examination showed that the right eye was totally paralyzed except for lateral eye movement (abduction). The right pupil was 3.0 mm and reacted normally to light. Visual acuity and fundoscopic exam was normal in both eyes. Extraocular movements of the left eye and the remainder of the neurologic examination were normal.

B) A 45-year-old male physician was admitted for evaluation of nocturnal fecal incontinence. Several episodes had occurred within the past month. Typically, he would awaken, without warning, to find his bed soiled. He had also complained of impotence for the past 5 years. His medical history was remarkable for long-standing diabetes mellitus which was insulin-dependent since he was 22 years old.

On examination BP 140/80, pulse 75 (supine); on standing, BP 90 systolic, pulse 75. Rectal examination was normal. There was a loss of pin and light touch appreciation in the legs in a stocking-glove distribution to the midcalf and decreased position and vibration sense in the feet; ankle jerks were absent. The remainder of the neurologic examination was normal.

NEUROANATOMICAL CLUE: Cross section of optic nerve.

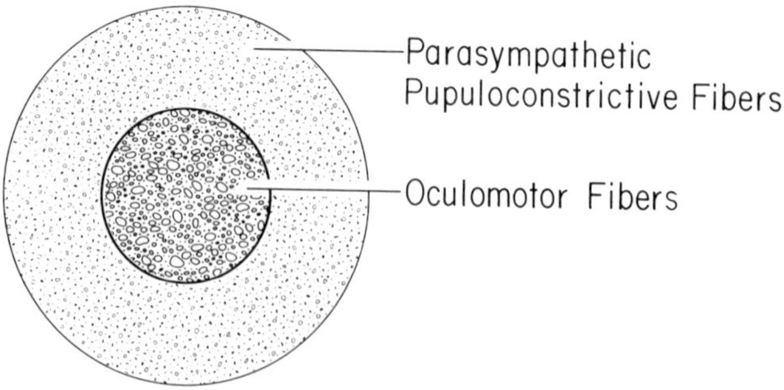

QUESTIONS:

1. What is the probable cause of diplopia in patient A? What laboratory test would confirm the diagnosis?

2. How does one distinguish between a third nerve palsy due to nerve infarction vs. one due to nerve compression? Could patient A have an intracerebral aneurysm?

3. What types of neuropathy does patient B have? What is their relationship, if any, to diabetes?

4. What treatment, if any, is available to patient A? patient B?

5. What additional neuropathic complications may occur in the patient with diabetes mellitus?

ANSWERS:

1. This patient has a <u>third nerve palsy</u>; the sudden onset of a third nerve palsy sparing the pupillary fibers is most likely due to diabetes mellitus. A fasting blood sugar or glucose tolerance test should confirm the diagnosis.

2. Infarction of the third nerve (diabetes, vasculitis, idiopathic) usually <u>spares the pupilloconstrictor fibers</u> which are on the outer perimeter of the nerve, i.e., vascular infarction occurs centrally (neuroanatomical clue). Thus, the pupil is of normal size and reacts; it is not large and unreactive as expected in third nerve palsy due to compression (aneurysm, herniation, tumor). <u>Note</u>: There have been reported cases of aneurysm with spared pupillary constriction.

3. This patient has an <u>autonomic neuropathy</u> as well as a polyneuropathy; both of these types of neuropathy are associated with diabetes mellitus.

4. There is no specific treatment for mononeuropathy due to diabetes; there is some evidence that further nerve injury may be prevented by careful medical management of the diabetic patient. For patients with orthostatic hypotension, elastic stockings and mineralocorticoid medication may be of benefit. Nocturnal incontinence may be helped by drugs which decrease peristalsis. Patients may also develop radiculopathy consisting of shooting pains, often confined to one dermatome; radiculopathy in the diabetic may simulate disc disease. In addition, diabetic amyotrophy may occur consisting of painful proximal muscle weakness and wasting; this diabetic complication is due to disease of the proximal motor nerves.

PEARLS:

1. <u>Elevated spinal fluid protein</u> is frequently due to diabetes.

2. <u>Sudden mononeuropathy</u> - think of diabetes.

3. Polyneuropathy in diabetics is associated with the accumulation of carbohydrates (sorbitol, inositol) in peripheral nerve.

4. Cervical spondylosis is more common in the patient with diabetes.

5. Diabetes may also be associated with a myelopathy, consisting of degeneration of the posterior columns of the spinal cord. These patients may have shooting pains and irregular, poorly reactive pupils, and the term "diabetic pseudotabes" describes the similarity of this condition to tabes dorsalis.

PITFALLS:

1. The polyneuropathy in diabetes may be painful. Tricyclics, Tegretol, and Dilantin have all been useful in the control of neuropathic pain in the diabetic.

2. Remember that hypoglycemia may produce focal neurologic deficits and all patients with insulin-dependent diabetes who develop sudden neurologic symptoms and signs should be treated initially for possible hypoglycemia.

3. Remember, the most common serious neurologic complication of diabetes mellitus is stroke.

REFERENCES

1. Asbury AK, Aldredge H, Herschberg R, et al: Ocular motor palsy and diabetes mellitus: a clinicopathological study. Brain 93:555, 1970.
2. Brown MJ, Asbury AK: Diabetic neuropathy. Ann Neurol 15:2, 1984.
3. Ewing DJ, Campbell IW, Clarke MF: The natural history of diabetic autonomic neuropathy. Quart J Med 49:95, 1980.
4. Kvinesdal B, et al: Imipramine treatment of painful diabetic neuropathy. JAMA 6;251:1727, 1984.
5. Raff MC, Asbury AK: Ischemic mononeuropathy and mononeuropathy multiplex in diabetes mellitus. N Engl J Med 279:17, 1968.
6. Spritz N: Nerve disease in diabetes mellitus. Med Clin North Am 62(4):787, 1978.

HODGKIN'S DISEASE, HEMIPARESIS, AND DEMENTIA

CASE 21: A 52-year-old man was admitted with a 1-week history of difficulty using his right arm. His family also reported that for 2 weeks his memory had been impaired and that he had been intermittently confused. Five years ago he was treated for Hodgkin's disease (stage 3B, nodular sclerosing type) with splenectomy, chemotherapy, and radiotherapy, and he had recently completed an additional course of local irradiation to the neck because of a local recurrence.

On examination, he was afebrile and appeared confused. Speech was fluent but dysphasic, with paraphasic errors and neologisms. Testing of extraocular movements revealed absent upgaze and sustained nystagmus on right lateral gaze. There was a right hemiparesis involving arm more than leg or face and bilateral extensor plantar responses. Limbs were ataxic and gait was staggering.

NEUROANATOMICAL CLUE: Enhanced CT scan.

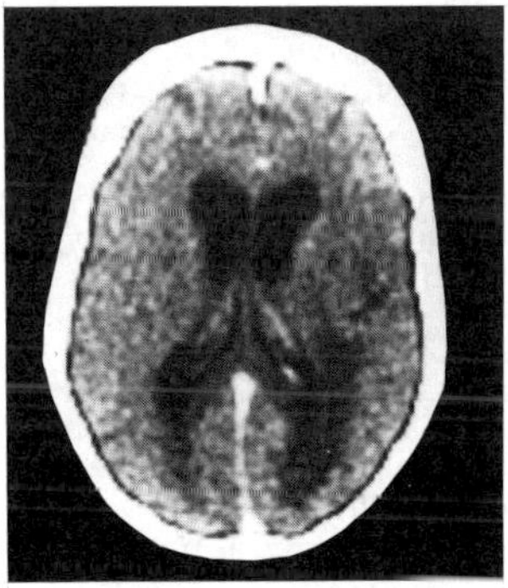

QUESTIONS:

1. Why is this clinical picture unlikely due to a metabolic disturbance?

2. What is your interpretation of the CT scan findings? Is this picture compatible with metastatic Hodgkin's disease?

3. What is your diagnosis?

4. What is the most definitive diagnostic test for this disease?

5. What is the prognosis? What treatment is appropriate?

ANSWERS:

1. Multiple focal symptoms and signs, including a right hemiparesis, absence of upgaze, and unilateral nystagmus were present. The neurologic signs of metabolic disorder are usually symmetric.

2. CT scan demonstrates multiple white matter lesions without mass effect and without enhancement following the injection of contrast dye. These lesions do not conform to vascular territories. In Hodgkin's disease, as in other tumors, mass effect and enhancement following the injection of contrast are usually seen.

3. Progressive, multifocal leukoencephalopathy (PML). PML is due to infection of oligodendrocytes by a papovavirus. Most cases of PML occur in patients with chronic malignancies (in particular, lymphomas and leukemias) and in patients with other illnesses causing immunosuppression (systemic lupus erythematosus, sarcoidosis, AIDS) or requiring chronic immunosuppressive drug therapy (for example, organ transplantation).

4. The definitive diagnostic test is a brain biopsy. Papovaviruses can be demonstrated by electron microscopy within oligodendrocytes.

5. The disease is typically relentlessly progressive and ends in death within 3-12 months following the onset of symptoms. Rarely, spontaneous remissions or a more chronic course occur. There is no proven effective therapy, although occasional reports suggest that cytarabine therapy may be effective in some patients.

PEARLS

1. Other conventional viruses which cause a chronic, multifocal neurologic disease are: measles virus (subacute sclerosing panencephalitis) and rubella (progressive rubella panencephalitis).

2. JC virus is the most important papovavirus responsible for PML. Serologic testing has shown that most individuals in the general population have had asymptomatic infection with JC virus at some time during their lives.

3. Creutzfeldt-Jakob disease, a "slow virus" infection generally does not preferentially occur in the immunosuppressed population and does not produce large lesions like those shown on the CT scan of this patient with PML.

4. In PML, typically no inflammation is present in brain or in spinal fluid.

PITFALL:

1. Multiple cerebral emboli (e.g., due to marantic endocarditis) in patients with underlying malignancy can give a clinical and CT scan picture similar to PML.

REFERENCES

1. Boudewijn Peters AC, Versteeg J, Bots GTAM, Boogerd W, Vielvoye GJ: Progressive multifocal leukoencephalopathy: immunofluorescent demonstration of simian virus 40 antigen in CSF cells and response to cytarabine therapy. Arch Neurol 37:497, 1980.
2. Sexton CR, Gailionas P Jr, Helderman JH, et al: Progressive multifocal leukoencephalopathy in a renal transplant recipient. Increased diagnostic sensitivity of computed tomographic scanning by double-dose contrast with delayed films. Am J Med 77:333, 1984.
3. Snider WD, et al: Neurological complications of acquired immune deficiency syndrome: Analysis of 50 patients. Ann Neurol 14:403, 1983.
4. Walker DL: Progressive multifocal leukoencephalopathy: An opportunistic viral infection of the central nervous system. In Handbook of Clinical Neurology, PJ Vinken, GW Bruyn (Eds). Vol. 34, Amsterdam, Elsevier-North-Holland, pp. 307, 1978.
5. ZuRhein GM, Chou SM: Particles resembling papovaviruses in human cerebral demyelinative disease. Science 148:1477, 1965.

UNILATERAL DEAFNESS

CASE 22: A 61-year-old woman complained of decreased hearing in the right ear. Her problem was progressive over a 1-year period and was associated with a chronic feeling of occipital "pressure." The patient denied vertigo, although she complained that "something is wrong with my head." She also complained of high-pitched tinnitus. She was otherwise in good health.

On examination, cranial nerve testing revealed normal visual acuity and sharp disc margins. There was nystagmus on right lateral gaze. Facial sensation was normal. Right-sided corneal stimulation evoked no blink response; left-sided stimulation resulted in a strong blink bilaterally. There was a moderate right facial weakness involving both the upper and lower portion of the face. When a vibrating tuning fork was applied to the forehead (Weber's test), the vibration was localized to the normal ear, suggesting a sensorineural hearing loss. The remainder of the examination was normal.

NEUROANATOMICAL CLUE: Localization of hearing loss.

The cochlea is the end-organ for hearing (as is the retina for vision). In the patient with deafness, it is important to ask: Is the hearing loss conductive (i.e., are impulses not reaching the cochlea) or sensorineural (i.e., is hearing loss due to cochlea or 8th nerve disease)?

Characteristics of conductive vs. sensorineural deafness:

Test	Normal Response	Conductive	Sensorineural
Midforehead tuning fork test (Weber)	Localized to both ears	Localized to affected ear	Localized to normal ear
Bone vs. air conduction test (Rinne)	Air > Bone	Bone > Air	Air > Bone

In patients with partial sensorineural deficits audiologic testing can help separate cochlea from nerve lesions.

Evaluation of partial sensorineural hearing loss: Cochlea versus nerve lesion:

Test	Cochlea	Nerve
Speech discrimination	Preserved	Reduced
Perceptions of a continuous tone	No decay	Decay
Perceptions of very loud sounds	Normal	Reduced

QUESTIONS:

1. What is Meniérè's disease?

2. What is tinnitus? What is its significance?

3. What is the significance of a reduced corneal response on right-sided stimulation in this woman? What is the significance of the right facial weakness?

4. What is the most likely diagnosis? What tests would you order?

ANSWERS:

1. Ménière's disease is an episodic hearing loss associated with vertigo and low-pitched tinnitus. Usually unilateral, Ménière's disease is an important cause of fluctuating hearing loss.

2. Tinnitus is any sensation of sound for which there is no source in the outside world. Tinnitus usually signifies disease of the middle or inner ear or of the 8th nerve.

3. A reduced right-sided corneal response with normal right-sided blinking on left-sided corneal stimulation suggests an abnormality of the afferent (5th cranial nerve) limb of the reflex. Right facial weakness involving both the upper and lower portions of the face indicates a lower motor neuron lesion of the 7th cranial nerve. Abnormalities of the 5th and 7th cranial nerves, in association with hearing loss, occur with lesions in the cerebellopontine angle.

4. Acoustic neuroma. Brainstem auditory evoked responses and a CT scan would be appropriate tests to support the clinical diagnosis.

PEARLS

1. Acoustic neuroma occurs commonly in patients with neurofibromatosis (von Recklinghausen's disease). A careful search for café-au-lait spots should be performed on all patients with suspected acoustic neuroma.

2. Otosclerosis, the most common cause of progressive deafness, is due to an overgrowth of bone within the middle ear.

3. Hereditary deaf-mutism, a dominantly inherited disorder, is due a congenital aplasia of the cochlea.

4. Occasionally, deafness can be a sign of vertebrobasilar disease. The internal auditory artery, which supplies the middle ear, is usually a branch of the anterior-inferior cerebellar artery.

5. Congenital deafness may follow rubella or syphilitic infection.

6. Hearing loss can occasionally occur from treatment with aminoglycoside antibiotics (streptomycin, gentamycin).

PITFALLS

1. Listen for bruits in the patient with tinnitus! The patient with physiologic tinnitus may hear a bruit or a hum secondary to atherosclerotic carotid artery disease or to a vascular malformation.

2. Most normal individuals will experience tinnitus when placed in quiet surroundings (physiologic tinnitus). Patients with depression may complain of physiologic tinnitus.

3. Hysterical hearing loss can be diagnosed by observing blinking to loud noises or by recording galvanic changes due to skin sweating induced by a loud sound (absent in true deafness).

REFERENCES

1. Adams RV, Victor M: Deafness, dizziness, and disorders of equilibrium. In Principles of Neurology, New York, McGraw-Hill, p. 190, 1981.
2. Dickins JR, et al: Ménière's disease 1978-1982. Am J Otol 5(2):137, 1983.
3. Lechtenberg R, Shulman A: The neurologic implications of tinnitus. Arch Neurol 41:718, 1984.
4. Mafee MF, Komar A, Valvassori GE, Dobben GD, Potter GD, Capek V: CT in the evaluation of the vestibulocochlear nerves and their central pathways. Evaluation of neurotologic disorders. Radiol Clin North Am 22:45, 1984.
5. Tinnitus (editorial). Lancet 1:543, 1984.
6. Wolfson RJ, et al: Vertigo. CIBA Clinical Symposia. 33(6), 1981.

VERTIGO AND DIZZINESS

CASE 23: A 62-year-old shopkeeper stayed home from work because of a "viral illness." After watching television, she stood up and walked toward the telephone. Suddenly, she felt the room spinning around her and she fell to the floor. She was nauseated and felt as if she had just stepped off a "merry-go-round." She lay perfectly still until the spinning sensation stopped. Then she stood up, only to be overcome again by severe vertigo; she fell down and vomited. She crawled to the phone and called her husband.

Later, examination in the emergency room demonstrated the following: BP 128/84, pulse 80 and regular. The patient lay perfectly still on the stretcher. There was no headache. Cranial nerve examination was normal except for mild rotatory nystagmus when the patient looked to the left. If the patient's head was abruptly turned in either direction, she became nauseated and said "the world is spinning." She grabbed the examining doctor for fear of falling from the stretcher. There was prominent rotatory nystagmus toward the left ear that diminished over 3-4 minutes. The remainder of the neurologic examination was normal.

QUESTIONS:

1. What is benign positional vertigo? How can one support this diagnosis at the bedside?

2. What features help distinguish between central and peripheral causes of vertigo?

3. What is the most likely etiology of this patient's dizziness?

4. What is the appropriate treatment? Prognosis?

5. Name some causes of dizziness in the elderly patient.

ANSWERS:

1. <u>Benign positional vertigo</u> (Bárány vertigo) is the most common cause of acute vertigo and consists of one or more episodes of vertigo without hearing loss. Vertigo and accompanying nystagmus can be seen at the <u>bedside</u> by moving the patient from a sitting position to a position with the head over the edge of the bed and turned 30 degrees to one side. The patient is then returned to the sitting position and the procedure is repeated with the head turned to the other side. Typically, one position will produce a brief recurrence of vertigo and nystagmus, which will decrease in severity with repeated testing. This illness is best treated by avoidance of the head positions which stimulate the symptoms.

2. Nystagmus of <u>peripheral</u> origin has these characteristic features on Bárány maneuver: a) it appears with a latency of several seconds; b) it is short-lived (less than 1 minute); c) it fatigues with repeated testing. Nystagmus of <u>central</u> origin has no latency, does not fatigue, and may last more than 1 minute. Vertical nystagmus or other brainstem signs or symptoms suggest central disease. Deafness with vertigo usually suggests peripheral disease.

3. <u>Labyrinthitis</u>. Dramatic onset with nausea, vomiting, and vertigo; no hearing loss. Spontaneously resolves within days to weeks.

4. Antihistamine drugs (Meclizine) and bedrest may help to control the vertigo and nausea.

5. <u>Multiple sensory deficits</u> (impaired hearing, vision loss, sensory loss) is an important cause of dizziness in the elderly. In addition, think of systemic (anemia or other metabolic), cardiovascular (Stokes-Adams), drug-induced, trauma, and vertebrobasilar causes. Cervical spine disease may also cause dizziness.

PEARLS:

1. Vertical nystagmus = brainstem dysfunction.

2. Vertigo + hearing loss = peripheral (end-organ or nerve disease).

3. Dizziness as an isolated symptom is usually not due to vertebrobasilar insufficiency.

4. Vertigo + tinnitus + deafness = Ménière's disease.

5. Nystagmus without vertigo is usually central (brainstem or central nervous system) in origin.

PITFALLS:

1. Chronic dizziness may be a sign of depression.

2. Dizziness and/or vertigo may occur with temporal lobe seizures.

3. Episodic dizziness or light-headedness may be due to a cardiac arrhythmia and may require Holter monitoring for diagnosis.

4. Acute vertigo in a hypertensive patient may be due to cerebellar hemorrhage or infarction and may mimic labyrinthitis.

REFERENCES

1. Brandt T, Daroff RB: The multisensory physiological and pathological vertigo syndromes. Ann Neurol 7:195, 1980.
2. Drachman D, Hart C: An approach to the dizzy patient. Neurology 22:323, 1972.
3. Fisher CM: Vertigo in cerebrovascular disease, Arch Otolaryngol 85:529, 1967.
4. Janetta PJ, Moller MB, Moller AR: Disabling positional vertigo. N Engl J Med 28:1700, 1984.
5. Rubenstein RL: Cerebellar infarction - a presentation of vertigo. The Laryngoscope 90:505, 1980.
6. Troost BT: Dizziness and vertigo in vertebrobasilar disease. Curr Concepts Cerebrovasc Dis 15(5)(6), 1979.
7. Wolfson RJ, et al: Vertigo. Ciba Symposia 33(6), 1981.

FACIAL WEAKNESS/FACIAL PAIN

CASE 24:

A) A 27-year-old man awoke with a left facial paralysis. One day earlier he had complained of pain behind his left ear. He also complained that noise from the left side seemed loud and unpleasant to him. He had previously been in excellent health, but had a strong family history of hypertension and cerebrovascular disease and he was fearful that he had suffered a stroke.

On examination, there was a complete facial paralysis on the left side involving both the upper and lower portions of the face; he was unable to close the left eye completely. There was reduced taste on the left anterior portion of the tongue. The remainder of the neurological examination was normal.

B) A 58-year-old woman had suffered for 10 years from attacks of pain across the left cheek. The pain was described as excruciating and knife-like. Each paroxysm of pain would last less than a second and would recur several times daily for periods of as long as 1 month. During these times, the pains would be triggered by chewing, brushing teeth, or touching the left side of the face and she would avoid going outside of her home for fear that wind might trigger the pain. The patient was chronically depressed and drank heavily, reportedly from fear of recurrent pain.

Neurological examination was completely normal.

QUESTIONS:

1. How does one differentiate between idiopathic facial palsy (Bell's palsy) and a stroke involving one side of the face?

2. What is the most important single laboratory test to be done in case A?

3. What would be the expected response to touching of the left cornea in case A? In case B?

4. For case A, what is the appropriate treatment? What is the prognosis?

5. What are delayed complications of facial palsy?

6. What is the diagnosis and appropriate treatment in case B?

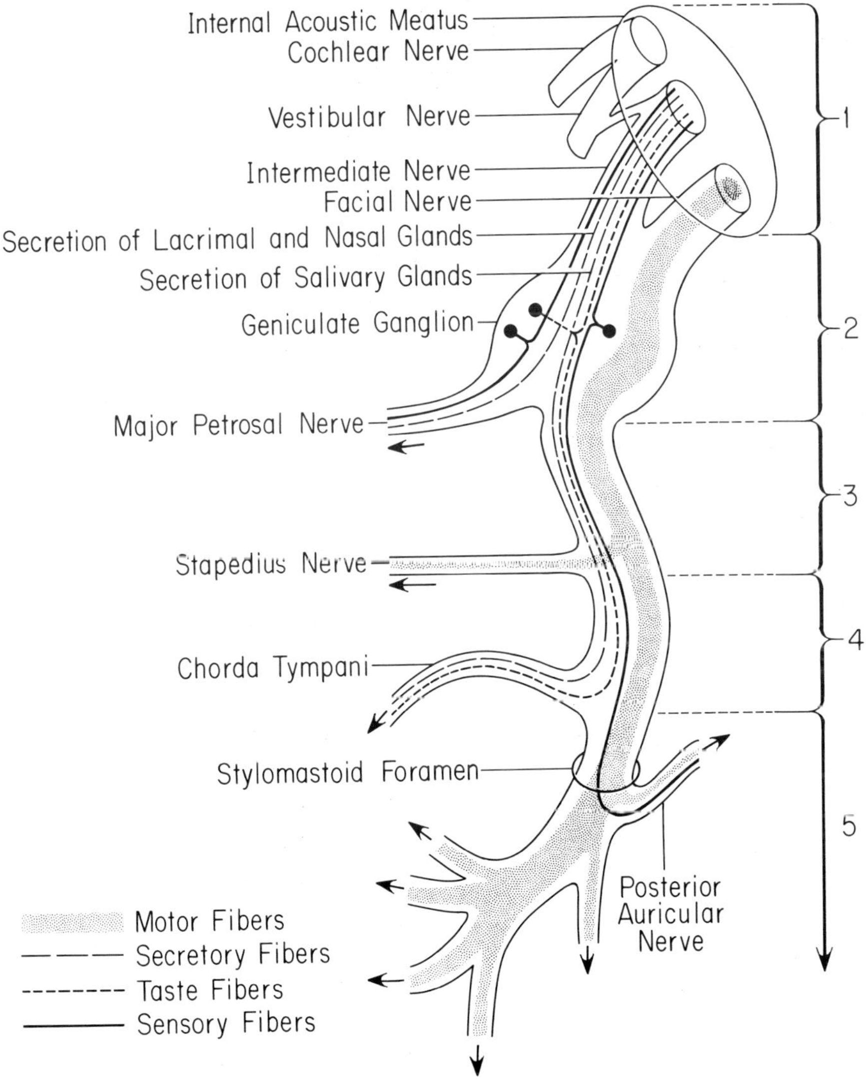

Diagram of Facial Nerve

ANSWERS:

1. Facial paralysis with abnormalities of taste sensation and with hyperacusis can only occur with a peripheral lesion of the 7th cranial nerve. This patient does not have a brainstem stroke because other symptoms and signs of brainstem disease are lacking. A stroke at levels above the brainstem would result in a contralateral facial paralysis which spares the upper portion of the face and would not affect taste or hearing.

2. Fasting blood glucose; there is an increased incidence of diabetes mellitus in patients with Bell's palsy.

3. In case A, the afferent (sensory) limb of the corneal reflex is intact, but there is a lesion of the efferent (motor) limb on the left side. Therefore, left corneal stimulation would result in a blink response on the right. In case B, one would expect the corneal reflex to be normal and, therefore, left-sided stimulation should result in a bilateral blink response.

4. Some authors recommend prednisone for early cases of Bell's palsy, although this is controversial. Treatment to prevent corneal ulceration (eye drops and lid closure during sleep) is essential. The prognosis is excellent and greater than 90% of patients will make a complete recovery within 6 months. Relapses are uncommon.

5. Late complications, due to abnormal reinnervation include involuntary eye closure or excess lacrimation (crocodile tears) during chewing.

6. Trigeminal neuralgia (tic douloureux). The most effective medical therapy is carbamazepine. Phenytoin may also be effective in some patients. In intractable cases, cryosurgery or electrocoagulation of a division of the trigeminal nerve may be required to control the symptoms. Trigeminal neuralgia may be caused by a neurofibroma or meningioma of the 5th cranial nerve, or by compression of the 5th nerve by a vertebral or basilar artery branch. The latter can be treated surgically with craniotomy and placement of a pleget under the 5th nerve.

PEARLS:

1. The etiology of Bell's palsy is unknown. Autoimmunity, vasculitis, or viral infection are suspected in most studies. In one study of epineural biopsies in patients with Bell's palsy, a high frequency of ischemic, hemorrhagic, or edematous changes were found.

2. Facial palsy, unilateral or bilateral, with associated facial swelling may be due to sarcoidosis.

3. There is an increased incidence of idiopathic facial palsy during pregnancy. In facial palsy of upper motor neuron or central origin, there is frequently good facial movement of the paralyzed side with emotional expression.

4. Ramsey-Hunt syndrome, due to herpes zoster of the 7th cranial nerve, consists of facial palsy and a vesicular eruption in the external auditory canal.

PITFALLS

1. Be sure to prevent corneal ulceration in patients with Bell's palsy with an eye patch and eye drops.

2. Bilateral or recurrent trigeminal neuralgia in a young person may be due to multiple sclerosis.

3. Beware of facial palsy, unilateral or bilateral, as an early sign of idiopathic polyneuritis (Guillain-Barré syndrome).

4. Beware of a diagnosis of trigeminal neuralgia in a patient with facial pain and objective sensory loss.

5. Carbamazepine may cause fatal agranulocytosis. Agranulocytosis is preceded by a period of reversible leukopenia. Periodic complete blood counts are mandatory in patients receiving carbamazepine.

REFERENCES

1. Abdour KA: Diagnosis and management of facial paralysis. N Engl J Med 307:348, 1982.
2. Fromm GH, Terrence CH, Maroon JC: Trigeminal neuralgia. Current concepts regarding etiology and pathogenesis. Arch Neurol 41:1204, 1984.
3. Horowitz SH: Isolated facial numbness: Clinical significance and relation to trigeminal neuropathy. Ann Intern Med 80:49, 1974.
4. Janetta P: Treatment of trigeminal neuralgia by micro-operative decompression. In Neurological Surgery, vol. 6, J. Youmans (Ed). Philadelphia, W.B. Saunders, pp. 589, 1982.
5. Kaplan JE, Greenspan JR, Bomgaars M et al: Simultaneous outbreaks of Guillain-Barré syndrome and Bell's palsy in Hawaii in 1981. JAMA 18:2635, 1983
6. Sade J: Pathology of Bell's palsy. Arch Otolaryngol 95:406, 1972.
7. Wepsic J: Tic-douloureux. N Engl J Med 288:680, 1973.

HEADACHES AND LEFT ARM WEAKNESS

CASE 25: A 36-year-old school teacher was evaluated for headaches and left arm weakness. The headaches began approximately 2 years previously, following an episode of severe coughing. Dull occipital pain had persisted on and off since that time. In addition, she had noted dull pain in the left hand during the past year. Six months ago she noted the onset of progressive numbness and weakness of the left hand and she reports that she is now unable to distinguish the temperature of bath water with her left hand. During the past month she also has found that her walking is "stiffer than usual." There have been no bowel or bladder abnormalities and her general health is otherwise well.

Examination was remarkable for mild thoracic kyphoscoliosis. Cranial nerve testing revealed a pupillary asymmetry (left 1 mm, right 3 mm). Both pupils were round and reactive. There was, in addition, a left ptosis. There was marked atrophy of all muscle groups in the left arm. There was complete loss of pain and temperature perception from C5 to T1 on the left and patchy abnormalities of pain and temperature sensation in the right forearm. Position and vibration perception were normal throughout. She was areflexic in the left arm and hyperreflexic in the right arm and in both legs, with moderate spasticity of both legs. Gait was mildly stiff-legged, but otherwise unremarkable.

QUESTIONS:

1. What is the significance of the dissociation between pain/temperature and position/vibration perception in this patient?
2. What is the most likely explanation for this patient's Horner's syndrome?
3. What is the most likely diagnosis?
4. What are the causes of this neurologic syndrome?
5. What workup is indicated?

ANSWERS:

1. Segmental loss of pain/temperature sensation with preservation of position/vibration sensation suggests a disease which is affecting the crossing pain and temperature fibers in the central portion of the spinal cord.

2. Horner's syndrome consists of ptosis, miosis, and facial hypohidrosis. In this case, this is most likely due to disease of the ipsilateral intermediolateral columns at C8-T1.

3. Segmental weakness with atrophy and dissociated sensory loss are most consistent with syringomyelia.

4. The majority of cases are idiopathic. Syringomyelia may complicate intramedullary or extramedullary spinal cord tumor (10-15%), may follow trauma, or may complicate chronic spinal arachnoiditis.

5. A myelogram will demonstrate swelling of the cervical spinal cord. A CT scan of the spinal cord may demonstrate syrinxes, especially in delayed views after a metrizamide myelogram. Magnetic resonance imaging may be the most sensitve of all tests for a syrinx.

PEARLS

1. Neck or head pain and stiffness of the legs are common early symptoms in syringomyelia.

2. Trauma or even coughing may precipitate signs of either syringomyelia or spinal cord tumor.

3. Idiopathic syringomyelia is associated with kyphoscoliosis as well as with a variety of abnormalities of the cervicomedullary junction, such as abnormal descent of cerebellar tonsils through the foramen magnum (type I Chiari malformation). Gardner has suggested that some cases may be due to poor CSF outflow through the fourth ventricle and transmission of ventricular pressure into the central canal.

4. CSF from patients with syringomyelia is usually normal, unless there is a spinal block, in which case one would then find increased protein. Fluid from within the syrinx in patients with idiopathic

syringomyelia is clear, but may have a yellow color and a high protein in patients with secondary syringomyelia from a spinal cord tumor.

5. Syringomyelia may be a late complication of severe spinal cord injury. In these patients an ascending spinal cord syndrome beginning at the level of the original trauma may develop years following the initial trauma.

6. The surgical treatment of syringomyelia has consisted of drainage of the upper end of the syrinx, opening of the 4th ventricular outflow tracts, or repair of the herniated cerebellar tonsils. In many patients, surgery has been followed by a temporary stabilization or improvement, although long-term controlled studies of surgery in this disease are lacking.

PITFALLS

1. Carefully examine all patients with unexplained spinal cord disease for neurocutaneous signs and symptoms. von Recklinghausen's disease and von Hippel Lindau syndrome are commonly associated with syringomyelia.

2. Question the diagnosis of syringomyelia in patients who have early incontinence. Fibers controlling bowel and bladder continence are located on the outer portion of the spinal canal and tend to be involved late in intramedullary spinal cord disease.

3. Suspect tumor in all patients with thoracic or lumbar syringomyelia.

REFERENCES

1. Barnett HJM, Foster JD, Hudgson P: *Syringomyelia*. Philadelphia, W.B. Saunders, 1973.
2. DiChiro G, Axelbaum SP, Schellinger D, Twigg HL, Ledley RF: Computerized axial tomography in syringomyelia. N Engl J Med 292:13, 1975.
3. Garcia-Uria J, Leunda G, Carrilo R, Bravo G: Syringomyelia: longterm results after posterior fossa decompression. J Neurosurg 54:380, 1980.
4. Gardner WJ: Hydrodynamic mechanism of syringomyelia: Its relationship to myelocele. J Neurol Neurosurg Psychiatry 28:247, 1965.
5. Pojunas K, Williams AL, Daniels DL, Haughton VM: Syringomyelia and hydromyelia: magnetic resonance evaluation. Radiology 153:679, 1984.
6. Williams B: A critical appraisal of posterior fossa surgery for communicating syringomyelia. Brain 101:223, 1978.

HEADACHE

<u>CASE 26</u>: A 54-year-old man had a 10-year history of headache. Some were characterized by unilateral throbbing pain with nausea, photophobia, and sound sensitivity; others by attacks of aphasia and right hemiparesis, followed by ipsilateral headache; and, others by lancinating pain in one or the other eye with ipsilateral nasal congestion and tearing of the eye. His general and neurological examinations between attacks were normal.

QUESTIONS:

1. Why is this patient unlikely to have a tumor causing his pain?

2. What different types of headache does this patient have?

3. What is the pathophysiological basis for migraine that explains its prodrome and headache phases?

4. What clinical features suggest cluster headache? Tension headache?

5. What is appropriate therapy for this patient?

ANSWERS:

1. The longstanding nature of this patient's headaches and the normal neurological examination argue against a tumor and for a benign cause.

2. This patient has three types of vascular headache: a) common migraine - unilateral throbbing pain with nausea; b) classic migraine - neurological prodrome (aura) preceding headache; c) cluster headache - unilateral eye pain, nasal congestion, and tearing.

3. Cerebral blood flow studies have shown decreased cerebral blood flow during the prodrome phase of migraine and vasodilatation with increased cerebral blood flow during the headache phase.

4. Cluster headache occurs almost exclusively in men and tends to recur at the same time every day for several weeks or months and then remit. During a cluster, patients may be awakened from sleep because of headache. Tension headache is usually bilateral, associated with a feeling of pressure rather than throbbing, and localized to the frontal and occipital regions. Tension headache is frequently associated with emotional stress or depression.

5. Ergot alkaloids (e.g., cafergot) taken during the prodrome may prevent the headache phase. Depending upon the frequency of attacks, propranolol may be effective as prophylaxis. For cluster headaches, daily prophylactic methysergide may be useful during the cluster period. Prednisone, lithium carbonate, and indomethacin have also been useful in cluster headache prophylaxis.

//Remember, migraine = headache, nausea, neurological disturbance. Any one of these symptoms may be absent//

PEARLS:

1. "Excruciating" headache and "sick" headaches are usually migrainous. "Marching" symptoms also suggest migraine, although they also occur with some focal seizure disorders. The "march" of migraine is typically slower (minutes) than the "march" of seizure (seconds).

2. Important treatable causes of headache in the elderly are glaucoma and temporal arteritis.

3. Repetitive single jabs of pain in the head or face are generally benign.

4. Women may experience an increase in migraine symptoms several days prior to each menstrual period. Premenstrual migraine may respond to salt restriction and diuretics.

5. "Cough" headache, although usually benign, may occur with brain tumor, cerebral malformation (Arnold-Chiari), or with other causes of raised intracranial pressure.

6. Scintillations consist of moving, flickering lights in one's visual field. Scintillations are characteristic of migraine.

PITFALLS:

1. Consider subarachnoid hemorrhage in patients with acute excruciating headache, whose headache is maximal at the onset.

2. Unilateral, recurrent throbbing headache which always occurs on the same side may be a symptom of an arteriovenous malformation.

3. Avoid ergot alkaloids in patients with severe neurological deficits (such as hemiplegia) during the migraine prodrome; these patients are best treated with prophylactic propranolol.

4. Think of chronic subdural hematoma in the alcoholic or elderly patient with chronic headache.

5. Remember that chronic headaches may be an important symptom of depression or other psychiatric disorder.

REFERENCES

1. Bartleson JD: Transient and persistent neurological manifestations of migraine. Stroke 15(2):383, 1984.
2. Caviness VS Jr, O'Brien P: Headache. N Engl J Med 302:446, 1980.
3. Dalessio DJ: Is there a difference between classic and common migraine? Arch Neurol 42:275, 1985.
4. Diamond S, Dalessio D: *The Practicing Physician's Approach to Headache*. Williams & Wilkins, Baltimore, 1982.
5. Diamond S, Medina JL: Headaches. CIBA Symposium 33(2), 1981.
6. Fisher CM: Transient migrainous accompaniments (TMAs) of late onset. Stroke 10:96, 1979.
7. Lance JW: Headache. Ann Neurol 10:1, 1981.
8. Sakai S, Myer JS: Regional, cerebral hemodynamics during migraine and cluster headaches measured by the Xenon inhalation method. Headache 18:122, 1978.
9. Ziegler DK: The headache symptom. How many entities? Arch Neurol 42:273, 1985.

SYMMETRIC WEAKNESS IN A YOUNG NURSE

CASE 27: A 28-year-old, black, female nurse was diagnosed as having systemic lupus erythematosus 3 years earlier on the basis of symptoms of photosensitivity, adenopathy, arthralgias, Raynaud's phenomenon, anti-DNA antibodies, and an elevated sedimentation rate. Most of her symptoms improved gradually without therapy and she was well until 6 months prior to admission when she developed progressive weakness. At first, her only symptoms were fatigue on walking long distances and difficulty climbing stairs, but the weakness then progressed to the point where she was unable to walk without a cane and was forced to stop working. During the past month, she noted for the first time weakness in her arms as well. There have been no sensory symptoms, fever, or pain, and her weakness has not fluctuated. There is no family history of neuromuscular or endocrine disease.

On examination, she was a thin woman in no distress. General physical examination was unremarkable. There was no rash. Extraocular movements and cranial nerve examination were normal. Muscle bulk was reduced, and there was symmetric weakness, more marked proximally, involving the lower limbs to a greater extent than the upper limbs. In the sitting position, she was just barely able to flex her hips against gravity. Tone was reduced, reflexes were present but reduced, and plantar responses were flexor. Sensory and cerebellar function were normal. With assistance, she was able to walk with a wobbly gait. Laboratory evaluation revealed normal thyroid and adrenal function and a sedimentation rate of 42 mm/hour. Serum creatinine phosphokinase (CPK) and aldolase were elevated. There was no response to an injection of intravenous edrophonium chloride (Tensilon).

QUESTIONS

1. What is the most likely cause of the symmetric weakness in this patient? What differential diagnosis should be considered?

2. What tests would you advise?

3. How should this patient be treated?

4. List some neurologic complications of systemic lupus erythematosus.

ANSWERS:

1. A myopathy. Symmetric, subacutely evolving muscle weakness in the absence of familial endocrine, metabolic, or toxic disease is most likely due to polymyositis. There is also an association between polymyositis and collagen vascular diseases. Other possibilities include sarcoidosis (granulomatous myopathy), infectious (toxoplasma, trichinosis, viral) causes and an unusual form of muscular dystrophy.

2. A) EMG. Findings characteristic of polymyositis consist of small polyphasic potentials, increased insertional activity, and fibrillation potentials. B) A muscle biopsy should also be performed. (Muscle biopsy in this patient showed inflammation with interstitial and perivascular mononuclear inflammatory cells, typical of polymyositis.)

3. Corticosteroids are considered to be the treatment of choice for polymyositis, although conclusive evidence for their efficacy is lacking. Immunosuppressive drugs, such as methotrexate, are used in patients who are corticosteroid resistant.

4. a) Cerebritis - altered mental function, seizures, focal neurological symptoms. These symtoms are thought to be due to cerebral vasculopathy (fibrinoid necrosis of small blood vessels) and infarction, although antineuronal antibodies have also been described; b) embolic strokes secondary to endocarditis (Libman-Sacks); c) mononeuritis multiplex - due to nerve infarction complicating vasculitis; d) symmetric sensory polyneuropathy.

PEARLS:

1. Dermatomyositis is distinguished from polymyositis by the presence in the former of an associated erythematous, scaly rash, which tends to localize over the extensor surfaces of joints, and by a heliotrope (violet, periorbital) rash.

2. Alcohol is an important cause of proximal myopathy.

3. Polymyositis is generally painless. This is in contrast to polymyalgia rheumatica, in which there is severe pain and little, if any, weakness.

4. An associated collagen vascular disease is present in up to one-half of patients with polymyositis and in most children with dermatomyositis.

5. Although both toxoplasmosis and Coxsackie virus have been associated with polymyositis-like illnesses, in most patients with polymyositis an infectious etiology cannot be found. The disease may be due to an autoimmune attack against muscle.

PITFALLS:

1. Do not perform a muscle biopsy at the site of a recent EMG! Artifacts, including muscle infarction and inflammation, may be present as a result of EMG studies.

2. Do not diagnose polymyositis if the muscle biopsy shows granulomas; this is most likely due to sarcoidosis.

3. All adults, particularly older adults, with dermatomyositis should have an extensive search for an underlying cancer. Adult dermatomyositis may be associated with malignancy and the symptoms of dermatomyositis precede the recognition of the tumor in two-thirds of those patients.

4. Steroid induced myopathy can mimic polymyositis, but muscle enzymes are usually not elevated in the former.

REFERENCES

1. Bohan A, Peter JB: Polymyositis and dermatomyositis. N Engl J Med 292:344-347, 403-407, 1975.
2. Bohan A, Peter JB, Bowman RL, Pearson CM: A computer-assisted analysis of 153 patients with polymyositis and dermatomyositis. Medicine (Baltimore) 56:255, 1977.
3. Whitaker JN: Inflammatory myopathy: A review of etiologic and pathogenetic factors. Muscle Nerve 5:573, 1982.
4. Tang TT, Sedmak GV, Siegesmund KA, McCreadie SR: Chronic myopathy associated with Coxsackie virus type A9: A combined electron microscopical and viral isolation study. N Engl J Med 292:608, 1975.
5. Johnson RT, Richardson EP: The neurological manifestations of systemic lupus erythematosus. Medicine (Baltimore) 47:337, 1968.

CHRONIC HEADACHE AND CSF PLEOCYTOSIS

CASE 28:

A) A 30-year-old electrical engineer developed increasingly severe headaches beginning 1 month prior to admission. Two weeks before admission he experienced intermittent vomiting. He was hospitalized following two episodes of confusion while at work. He had also noted a low-grade fever on several occasions during the past month.

Examination revealed an afebrile, disoriented and agitated young man who was intermittently able to answer simple questions. General examination was unremarkable. His neck was supple. Neurological examination revealed roving eye movements and normal cranial nerve function. He moved all limbs with good strength. Reflexes were 2+ and symmetrical and plantar responses were flexor.

Serum sodium was 125 mmol and serum osmolarity 263 mOsm/liter. Complete blood count and SMA 20 were normal. A CT scan revealed moderate ventricular enlargement. Lumbar puncture revealed slightly cloudy fluid with an opening pressure of 300 mm H_2O, 92 lymphocytes, and 10 neutrophils/mm^3. CSF glucose was 26 mg% and protein 408 mg%.

B) A 47-year-old married painter was admitted for evaluation of headaches, episodes of shaking movements of his right arm, and slurred speech. His work involved painting and restoration of interior and exterior building surfaces. His past history included throbbing headaches when he was a teenager, but was otherwise negative.

Examination was unremarkable, except for a temperature of 100.8°F and mild nuchal rigidity. EEG, CT scan, and left carotid arteriogram were normal, but a spinal tap revealed an opening pressure of 220 mm, 81 lymphocytes, 21 red cells, protein 95 mg%, and sugar 28 mg%. CSF gram stain looked normal. When the correct diagnosis was established, appropriate therapy led to complete resolution of all symptoms.

QUESTIONS:

1. Both patients have chronic meningitis. What are the major causes of this syndrome?

2. What are the characteristic cerebrospinal fluid (CSF) findings in chronic meningitis?

3. What is the most likely diagnosis in case A? How should this patient be treated?

4. An India ink stain of the CSF in case B revealed the following:

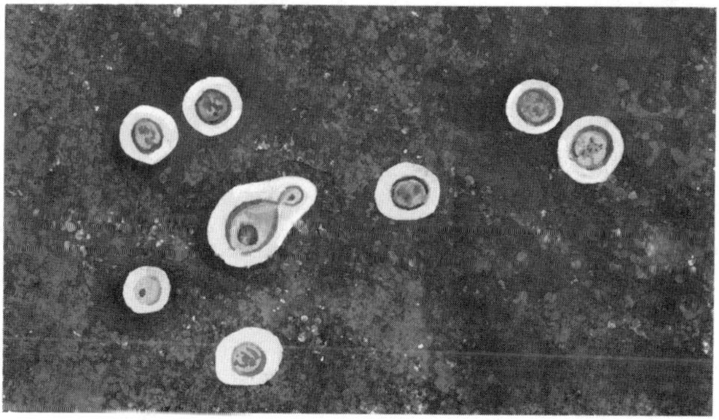

   a) What is your diagnosis? b) How can it be confirmed? c) What is the optimal therapy?

5. What is the normal CSF glucose value? What conditions cause reduced CSF glucose (hypoglycorrhachia)?

ANSWERS:

1. Tuberculosis, fungi, syphilis, meningeal carcinomatosus, systemic diseases (sarcoidosis, Bechet's disease, lupus erythematosus).

2. Increased opening pressure, CSF pleocytosis with mononuclear predominance, elevated protein, and low sugar.

3. This patient had <u>tuberculous meningitis</u>. Antituberculous therapy is usually instituted pending definitive diagnosis in patients with unexplained subacute meningoencephalitis with hydrocephalus and appropriate CSF profile (lymphocyte predominance, decreased glucose, and elevated protein). Therapy consists of isoniazid and rifampicin; some centers add a third drug in addition, either streptomycin or ethambutol. Therapy is usually continued for 18-24 months.

4. a) <u>Cryptococcal meningitis</u>. The picture is an India ink stain demonstrating the thick capsule of cryptococci. b) <u>Cryptococcal antigen</u> can be detected in CSF by a latex agglutination test in 95% of patients, and the organism can usually be cultured from CSF. c) <u>Amphotericin B</u> is the treatment of choice. Flucytosine may be added to amphotericin. In patients who do not respond rapidly to intravenous therapy, direct intrathecal administration may be required to sterilize the CNS.

5. <u>CSF glucose levels are approximately two-thirds of the blood glucose level</u>. Reduced CSF glucose is seen in bacterial, fungal, and tuberculous meningitis, meningeal carcinomatosus, subarachnoid hemorrhage, and sarcoidosis. Occasionally, viral CNS infections (mumps, herpes simplex virus, and eastern equine encephalitis) can also reduce the CSF glucose content.

PEARLS:

1. The "immunocompromised host" is a good candidate for fungal meningitis, although fungal meningitis may also occur in normal adults (as, for example, case B).

2. Tuberculous meningitis is usually caused by the breakdown of an asymptomatic CNS tuberculoma.

3. Approximately 20% of patients with tuberculous meningitis have no clinical or radiologic evidence of extrameningeal tuberculosis.

4. Empirical therapy for tuberculous meningitis should be initiated in patients with a high index of suspicion while cultures are pending.

5. Tuberculosis may cause a transient, aseptic meningitis followed by complete recovery ("serous tuberculous meningitis").

PITFALLS:

1. Think of hydrocephalus when dementia or change in level of consciousness develops in a patient with chronic meningitis. Hydrocephalus, due to blockage of CSF circulation by exudate, was a complication of tuberculous meningitis in case A.

2. Untreated chronic meningitis has a high morbidity and mortality. Expeditious diagnosis is essential.

3. When confronted with sudden paraplegia in a young person, think of tuberculosis as a possible cause; spinal X-rays may disclose bony lesions of tuberculosis (Pott's disease).

4. Stroke may be a complication of tuberculous or fungal meningitis and is secondary to arterial involvement by vasculitis with secondary thrombosis.

REFERENCES

1. Bennett JE, et al.: A comparison of amphotericin B alone and combined with flucytosine in the treatment of cryptococcal meningitis. N Engl J Med 301:126, 1979.
2. Diamond RD, Bennett JE: Prognostic factors in cryptoccal meningitis. A study in 111 cases. Ann Intern Med 80:176, 1974.
3. Ellmer JJ Bennett JE, Dismukes WE, Dumar J, et al.: Chronic meningitis. Medicine (Baltimore)55:341, 1976.
4. Fallon RJ: The treatment of tuberculous meningitis. J Antimicrob Chemother 4:1, 1978.
5. Heas EJ, Madhavan P, Quinn EL, Cox F, Fisher E, Burch K: Tuberculous meningitis in an urban general hospital. Arch Int Med 137:1518, 1977.
6. Olson ME, Chernik ML, Posner JB: Infiltration of the leptomeninges by systemic cancer. Arch Neurol 30:122, 1974.

7. Salaki M et al: Fungal and yeast infections of central nervous system. Medicine 63(2):108, 1984.
8. Tandon PN: Tuberculous meningitis. In _Handbook of Clinical Neurology_, PJ Vinken and GW Bruyn (Eds). Vol. 33, Infections of the Nervous System, Part 1. Amsterdam, Elsevier-North/Holland, 1978.
9. Traub M, Colchester ACF, Kingsley DPE, Swash M: Tuberculosis of the central nervous system. Quart J Med 53:81, 1984.
10. Zeluff W: Chronic meningitis - benign and malignant forms. Heart and Lung 9(3):534, 1980.

HEADACHE AND INTERMITTENT CONFUSION

CASE 29: You are asked to see a 37-year-old woman, a successful corporate lawyer, because of increasing headaches which began approximately 1 month ago. She first noted headache several days after returning from a ski trip with her husband and two children. The headaches are bifrontal, throbbing, and increasing in severity. During the past week she has awakened from sleep on several occasions with headache and vomiting. In addition, her husband describes her as more apathetic and less "sharp" at work than usual. One week ago she saw a local physician who prescribed Valium. There have been no visual, motor, or sensory complaints. She is not on any medications, has no other medical illnesses, and has suffered no recent trauma.

On examination, she was tearful and complained of severe steady headache and an inability to sleep for several days. She relied on her husband for most of the details of her illness. On several occasions, she did not respond to questions asked directly to her and the questions had to be repeated. There was no aphasia, but detailed mental status testing was impossible because of her agitated state. Examination of the optic fundi revealed an absence of venous pulsations and blurring of the disc margins. The remainder of the cranial nerve examination was normal. There was a mild pronator drift of the right arm, but power was otherwise normal. There was reflex asymmetry (3/5 on the right; 2/5 on the left) and plantar responses were flexor on the left and equivocal on the right. Tone, sensory, and cerebellar examinations were within normal limits, and her gait was normal. A CT scan was performed.

QUESTIONS:

1. What is your interpretation of the CT scan?

2. What is the etiology of this condition?

3. Name the predisposing conditions or medical illnesses that are associated with this disease.

4. What is the appropriate therapy?

NEUROANATOMICAL CLUE:

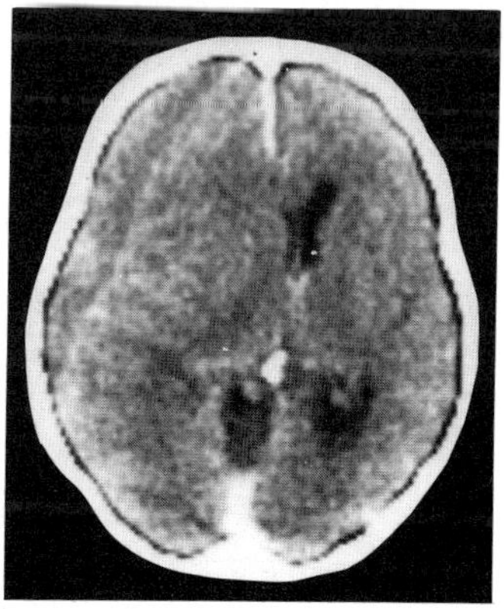

ANSWERS:

1. The scan shows a large, left-sided, isodense, chronic subdural hematoma. On the nonenhanced scan, the subdural hematoma itself was not visible because of its isodense character, but a shift of the lateral ventricles due to mass effect was seen. With contrast enhancement, the membranous wall of the subdural can be seen and the size of the subdural collection is clearly outlined.

2. Subdural hematomas are caused by tearing of subdural veins and by bleeding into the subdural space. The subdural collection may then enlarge over subsequent weeks; the mechanisms which cause subdural hematomas to enlarge are unknown.

3. Trauma is the most important predisposing condition for acute subdural hematoma, but in patients with chronic subdural hematoma a history of trauma may be absent in up to 50% of patients; frequently, the trauma is minor. This patient, in retrospect, remembered several falls during her ski vacation, although none appeared at the time to be serious. Other predisposing conditions include anticoagulation, renal failure and dialysis, epilepsy, and alcohol or other drug abuse.

4. The treatment for symptomatic, chronic subdural hematomas is surgical evacuation. In patients with small, stable subdural hematomas, or in those for whom surgery is contraindicated, medical management with corticosteroids and dehydrating agents (mannitol) may be successful. In this patient surgical evacuation was performed with excellent results.

PEARLS:

1. Subdural hematoma typically produces changes in the level of consciousness out of proportion to focal neurologic signs and symptoms. Thus, typical symptoms include headache (75%), slowness of thought, confusion, and apathy. Complete hemiplegia, aphasia, or homonymous hemianopsia is rare in patients with subdural hematoma.

2. An important clue to subdural hematoma is the presence of fluctuating levels of consciousness.

3. The differential diagnosis of subdural hematoma, particularly in the elderly, includes cerebrovascular disease (onset of symptoms is usually acute) and metabolic or drug-related causes (rarely have focal neurologic findings).

4. The CT scan is the most important diagnostic test for subdural hematoma. Rarely, an isodense subdural hematoma is missed on CT scan and in those patients angiography may be necessary.

PITFALLS:

1. Think of the possibility of subdural hematoma in the appropriate clinical setting. A large proportion of subdural hematomas are missed initially, even in hospitalized patients.

2. Headache which awakens a patient from sleep often signifies serious central nervous system disease (exception, cluster headache).

3. Beware of the diagnosis of depression or hysteria as an explanation of any medical symptom of recent onset. This patient's symptoms were initially felt to be of functional origin.

4. Think about the diagnosis of subdural hematoma in any patient on anticoagulation who develops unexplained headache, particularly if other neurologic symptoms are present.

REFERENCES

1. Cameron MM: Chronic subdural haematoma; a review of 114 cases. J Neurol Neurosurg Psychiatry 41:834, 1978.
2. Dronfield MW, Mead GM, Langman MJS: Survival and death from subdural hematoma on medical wards. Postgrad Med J 53:57, 1977.
3. McKissock W, Richardson A, Blume WH: Subdural haematoma. A review of 389 cases. Lancet 1:1365, 1960.
4. Moster ML, et al: Chronic subdural hematoma with transient neurological deficits: A review of 15 cases. Ann Neurol 14:539, 1983.
5. Seelig JM, et al: Traumatic acute subdural hematoma. N Engl J Med 304:1511, 1981.
6. The recognition of chronic subdural haematoma (editorial). Lancet 2:449, 1979.

SUDDEN HEADACHE AND STIFF NECK IN A COLLEGE STUDENT

CASE 30: A 20-year-old student was admitted for evaluation of "the worst headache of my life." Twelve days earlier, while out with friends, she noted the sudden onset of a severe headache with nausea; she was brought to a local emergency ward, where a diagnosis of "tension headache" was made. Her headache subsided over several days and she returned to her usual state of good health. On the morning of admission, while sitting on the toilet, she developed a sudden recurrent headache "even worse than the last one" with vomiting and she thought she might have lost consciousness momentarily. Apparently, a roommate heard her scream and brought her to the emergency room.

Examination demonstrated a young woman in excruciating pain, lying flat on the examination table, avoiding any movements. Blood pressure 160/100; pulse 120. There was marked nuchal rigidity. Retinal examination revealed bilateral subhyaloid hemorrhages around the optic discs. Although intermittently drowsy, her mental status examination and detailed neurological examination was otherwise normal.

QUESTIONS:

1. What is your diagnosis? What laboratory tests should be ordered?

2. What are the common presenting features of this condition?

3. How are patients with this illness classified?

4. What are the two major complications of this disease?

5. What is the appropriate medical therapy? Surgical therapy?

NEUROANATOMICAL CLUE:

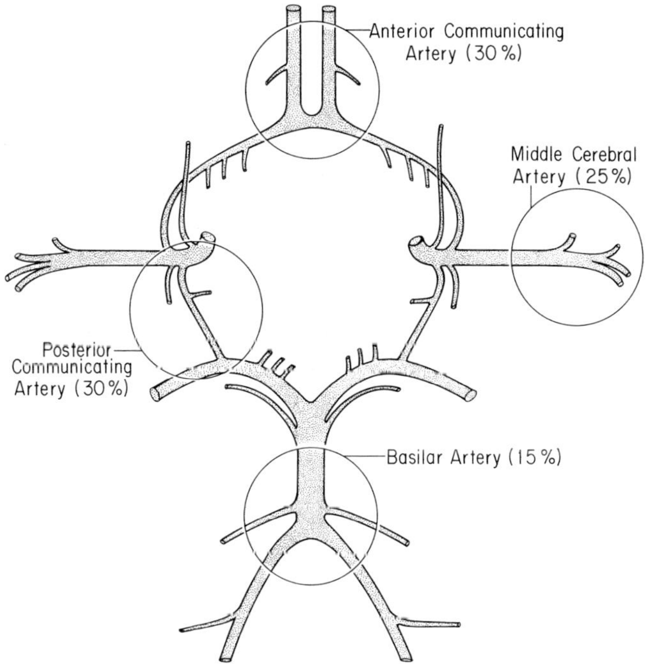

ANSWERS:

1. Subarachnoid hemorrhage. A CT scan confirmed the presence of subarachnoid bleeding; if a CT scan is not available, a lumbar puncture should be performed. This patient likely had two bleeds from the same saccular ("Berry") aneurysm within a 12-day period.

2. Acute onset of severe headache. The vast majority of patients with subarachnoid hemorrhage have not had previous symptoms from aneurysms. Rarely, patients complain of headache preceding aneurysm rupture, or occasionally an expanding aneurysm may produce symptoms due to compression of adjacent structures.

3. Classification of acute subarachnoid hemorrhage: grade 1 - headache only; grade 2 - some drowsiness or clouding of consciousness is present; grade 3 - definite focal neurological signs or major alterations in consciousness are present; grade 4 - severe focal deficits (hemiplegia, aphasia); grade 5 - coma. This patient would be classified as grade 2.

4. a) Spasm of cerebral vessels adjacent to site of rupture - develops between day 4 and 14 following subarachnoid hemorrhage and may result in ischemia and stroke. The risk of symptomatic spasm is directly related to the volume of blood in the subarachnoid space. b) Rebleeding - although uncommon within the first 48 hours following subarachnoid hemorrhage, there is a high risk of rebleeding subsequently; 40% of patients rebleed within 2 months following a subarachnoid hemorrhage, and many of those patients will rebleed within 3 weeks. Most deaths due to subarachnoid hemorrhage are due to rebleeding, rather than due to the effects of the initial hemorrhage.

5. Acute medical therapy includes bed rest, sedation, and adequate analgesia; blood pressure should be controlled and hypotension avoided. Calcium blockers (nimodipine) have been shown to decrease the risk of spasm in grade 1 patients and many centers advocate antifibrinolytic therapy (epsilon-amino-caproic acid) to prevent rebleeding, although this remains controversial. Surgical treatment consists of clipping of the aneurysms and most surgeons advise waiting 10-14 days following subarachnoid hemorrhage before surgery is attempted.

PEARLS:

1. In patients with subarachnoid hemorrhage not treated surgically, 10-year follow-up has revealed a steady incidence of late rebleeding of approximately 3% per year.

   NEUROANATOMICAL CLUE: Location and frequency of saccular aneurysyms.

2. Some neurological syndromes associated with subarachnoid hemorrhage may give a clue to the vessels which have bled. Thus, a third nerve palsy is seen with aneurysms of the posterior communicating artery, bilateral leg weakness with anterior communicating artery aneurysm, and aphasia and/or hemiplegia with middle cerebral artery aneurysm.

3. There is an increased risk of saccular aneurysm and of subarachnoid hemorrhage in patients with polycystic kidney disease and with aortic coarctation.

4. "Nonlocalizing" symptoms of subarachnoid hemorrhage may include a 6th nerve palsy and transient amnesia.

5. Subarachnoid hemorrhage is rare before the age of 10 years and occurs with increasing frequency with each succeeding decade. There are 28,000 new cases of subarachnoid hemorrhage in the United States yearly.

PITFALLS:

1. In all conditions which result in meningeal irritation, neck rigidity tends to disappear as the level of consciousness decreases.

2. Progressive hydrocephalus due to blockage of CSF resorption by blood may occur 2-4 weeks following subarachnoid hemorrhage; think of secondary hydrocephalus in patients who deteriorate during this period.

3. A brisk leukocytosis may occur in the CSF 48 hours following subarachnoid hemorrhage and does not necessarily indicate infection in these patients.

4. The optic chiasm syndrome (bitemporal hemianopsia) may be due to mass effect from an aneurysm of the internal carotid artery; for this reason, angiogram should be performed in all patients prior to surgery for suspected pituitary adenoma.

5. A normal CT scan does not exclude subarachnoid hemorrhage - perform a lumbar puncture in subarachnoid hemorrhage suspects who have negative CT scans.

REFERENCES

1. Adams HP Jr, Kassell MF, Torner JC, Mibbelink DW, Sahs AL: Early management of aneurysmal subarachnoid hemorrhage: a report of the cooperative aneurysm study. J Neursurg 54:151, 1981.
2. Allen GS, Ahn HS, Preziosi TJ, et al.: Cerebral arterial spasm, a controlled trial of nimodipine in patients with subarachnoid hemorrhage. N Engl J Med 308:619, 1983.
3. Chyette D, Sundt TM Jr: Cerebral vasospasm after subarachnoid hemorrhage. Mayo Clin Proc 59:498, 1984.
4. Drake CG: Management of cerebral aneurysm. Stroke 12:273, 1981.
5. Fisher CM, Kistler JP, Davis JM: Relation of cerebral vasospasm to subarchnoid hemorrhage visualized by computerized tomographic scanning. Neurosurgery 6:1, 1980.
6. Heros R, Kistler JP: Intracranial arterial aneurysms: An update. Curr Concepts Cerebrovasc Dis 18(1):1, 1983.
7. Heros R, Zervas N: Subarachnoid hemorrhage. Ann Rev Med 34:367, 1983.
8. McKissock W, Paine KW, Walsh LS: An analysis of the results of treatment of ruptured intracranial aneurysms: a report of 722 consecutive cases. J Neurosurg 17:762, 1962.
9. Review of subarachnoid hemorrhage in Seminars in Neurology, Vol 4, No. 3, Sept. 1984.
10. Sundt TM Jr, Whisnant JP: Subarachnoid hemorrhage from intracranial aneurysms: surgical management and natural history of disease. N Engl J Med 299:116, 1978.
11. Vermeulan M, Lindsay KW, Murray GD, et al: Anti-fibrinolytic treatment in subarachnoid hemorrhage. N Engl J Med 311:432, 1984.

COMA WITHOUT FOCAL SIGNS

CASE 31: A 53-year-old, married woman was found comatose in bed. Her past history was negative except for mild hypertension. She had had some recent adversity in her business, but had not seemed depressed. Examination found a deeply comatose woman unresponsive to voice or deep pain. Blood pressure, 90/50; pulse, 110, regular; respirations, 20 and regular. General physical examination was normal. Pupils were small and reactive to light. There were no eye movements with doll's head maneuver, no response to ice water calorics, no corneal reflexes, no gag. She was areflexic and toes were downgoing. Spinal tap was normal. EEG showed bilateral fast activity superimposed on slow background rhythms, but no focal abnormality.

QUESTIONS:

1. What is the most likely general cause of this patient's coma? Why?
2. What are the important steps in the initial management of the patient with coma of unknown cause?
3. What is decorticate posturing? What does it usually signify? Decerebrate posturing?
4. Name some rapidly reversible causes of coma if diagnosed early.
5. Brain metabolism may fail because of exogenous toxins, endogenous toxins, or because of a lack of energy sources. Name some causes of coma in each category.

ANSWERS:

1. A metabolic-toxic cause. The causes of coma can be divided into three pathophysiologic categories: toxic-metabolic, supratentorial lesions, and infratentorial lesions. Because of the symmetry of neurologic signs and the presence of normal pupillary responses and regular respirations in the absence of other brainstem function, a toxic metabolic cause was most likely. As it turned out, this patient left a suicide note and took a barbiturate overdose.

2. Initial management of the comatose patient includes assuring ventilation and oxygenation, maintaining circulation, and stopping seizures if present. Blood samples should be drawn for CBC and chemistries and for a toxic screen. In most instances, the patient should then be given sequential intravenous injections of thiamine, glucose, and naloxone and the clinical response, if any, to each injection should be observed.

3. Decorticate posturing indicates damage to the hemispheres or diencephalon; decerebrate posturing is seen with destructive lesions to the midbrain and upper pons. Both toxic/metabolic causes of coma and destructive brain lesions can result in decorticate and decerebrate posturing.

4. Hypoglycemia, narcotic drug overdose, hypercapnia, diabetic ketoacidosis, myxedema, Addisonian crisis, electrolyte imbalance (especially hyponatremia).

5. Exogenous - drugs and toxins; endogenous - uremia, hepatic failure; decreased energy source - hypoxia, hypoglycemia.

PEARLS:

1. The goal of the evaluation of the comatose patient is to find a treatable cause.

2. In metabolic coma, eye signs may give a clue to the etiology. For example: normal pupillary responses but absent eye movements = barbiturates; pinpoint pupils = opiates; fixed and dilated pupils = atropine.

3. In comatose patients, ice water calorics are performed to assess function of the vestibular-ocular systems in the pons and midbrain; in patients with full eye movements on doll's head maneuver, caloric testing is unnecessary.

4. Look for clues to cause of coma in general physical exam, e.g., breath odor, bruises, neck stiffness, breathing pattern, evidence of renal or hepatic disease.

5. The EEG can be helpful in evaluating comatose patients: The EEG a) shows bilateral slowing in metabolic coma; b) is normal in "psychogenic" coma; c) may show "beta" or fast activity with drug overdosage; and d) is isoelectric (flat) in brain dead patients.

PITFALLS:

1. Glucose given to malnourished patients without concomitant thiamine will precipitate or worsen Wernicke's encephalopathy.

2. Massive intracerebral hemorrhage and bilateral cerebral hemisphere infarction can simulate "metabolic" coma.

3. Hypoglycemia can present with seizures and focal signs.

4. Sedative poisoning and hypothermia may result in absent electrocerebral activity on EEG that does not necessarily signify brain death. Brainstem auditory evoked study is useful in such cases.

REFERENCES

1. Caronna J, Simon RP: The comatose patient: A diagnostic approach and treatment. Int Anesthesiol Clin 17:3, 1979.
2. Levy DE, Bates D, Caronna J, et al: Prognosis in nontraumatic coma. Ann Intern Med 94:293, 1981.
3. Levy DE, Caronna JJ, et al: Predicting outcome from hypoxic-ischemic coma. JAMA 253:1420, 1985.
4. Plum F, Posner J: Diagnosis of Stupor and Coma, 3rd edition. Philadelphia, F.A. Davis, 1982.

FACIAL NUMBNESS AND ATAXIA

CASE 32: A 64-year-old, married man with known hypertension awoke to find that his gait was unsteady and that the left side of his face felt numb. There was no headache, paralysis, or diplopia. On examination, his blood pressure was 160/100; he was alert and had fluent speech, but his voice was hoarse. He had a left ptosis, miotic left pupil, and decreased pin and temperature appreciation of the left face and right side of his body. There was no nystagmus on gaze to the left. He had a gait ataxia with falling toward the left side and ataxia of his left limbs. Strength and reflexes were normal. CT scan, spinal tap, and EEG were normal.

QUESTIONS:

1. What type of stroke did this patient have (thrombosis, embolus, hemorrhage)? Where was it located? What is the likely etiology?

2. What is the appropriate treatment? What is the prognosis?

3. a) What is the most common associated risk factor for this stroke syndrome? b) Name three other risk factors for stroke.

4. Is anticoagulation indicated in this patient?

5. Name an analogous posterior circulation stroke syndrome in which hearing loss and tinnitus are hallmarks. What other characteristic features are present?

NEUROANATOMICAL CLUE:

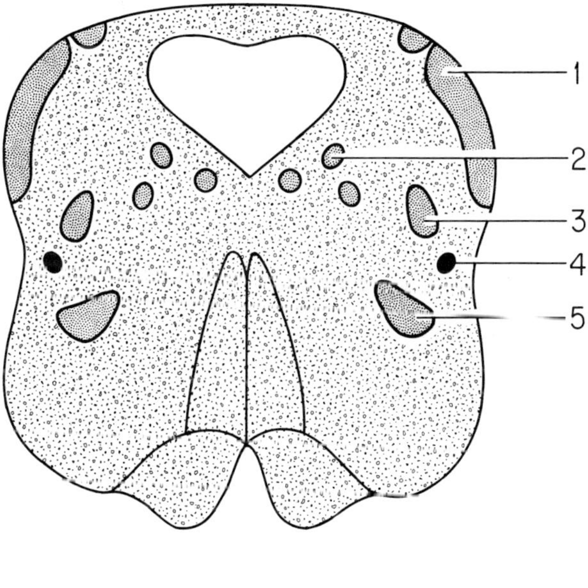

Label the numbered structures in the diagram of the medulla and relate each structure to a symptom or sign that the patient showed.

ANSWERS:

1. Thrombotic stroke affecting the left lateral medulla (Wallenberg's syndrome). In the majority of cases this syndrome is due to thrombotic occlusion of the ipsilateral vertebral artery intracranially. Some cases are due to occlusion of the posterior inferior cerebellar artery (PICA) itself.

   NEUROANATOMICAL CLUE:

   1. Inferior cerebellar peduncle - ataxia.
   2. X nerve nucleus - hoarseness.
   3. Descending tract of V - numb face.
   4. Sympathetics - Horner's syndrome.
   5. Lateral spinothalamic tract - numbness of the body (contralateral).

2. Supportive, with gradual treatment of associated hypertension if present. Most patients survive and do not develop other posterior circulation strokes. There is a relatively benign form of the lateral medullary syndrome seen in young adults following exercise which has an excellent long term prognosis.

3. a) Hypertension. b) Other risk factors for stroke include diabetes mellitus, underlying heart disease (particularly atrial fibrillation and rheumatic valve disease), and transient ischemic attacks. Obesity, cigarette smoking, and physical inactivity may be additional risk factors for stroke, but the data are inconclusive.

4. No; this is a completed thrombotic stroke for which anticoagulation is not indicated and could potentially prove harmful. However, some physicians would put a patient such as this on antiplatelet agents. In the posterior circulation, anticoagulation is reserved for partial large vessel syndromes (e.g., partial basilar thrombosis), strokes thought to be of embolic origin (e.g., "top of the basilar" syndrome), or "stroke in evolution."

5. Lateral inferior pontine syndrome (occlusion of anterior inferior cerebellar artery). Horizontal and vertical nystagmus and vertigo due to involvement of vestibular nerve or nucleus, facial paralysis, ataxia, impaired sensation of the face on side of the lesion and of the body on the side contralateral to the lesion.

PEARLS:

1. Sudden hoarseness -- think of medullary or vocal cord lesion.
2. Sudden ataxia without weakness -- think of a lesion in cerebellum or vestibular system or in their connections.
3. Crossed cranial nerve and long tract signs = brainstem lesion; bilateral motor and sensory signs = brainstem or spinal cord lesion.
4. Elevated blood pressure should be lowered vigorously in hemorrhagic stroke, but very cautiously in thrombotic stroke.
5. Do not anticoagulate completed thrombotic strokes!

PITFALLS:

1. Aspiration is a common complication of the lateral medullary syndrome because of dysphagia due to involvement of the tenth nerve nucleus. Keeping the patient NPO until gag and swallowing function return is mandatory.
2. Clinically significant cerebellar infarction may accompany the lateral medullary syndrome and can lead to cerebellar swelling, brainstem compression, and death unless surgically relieved.
3. Posterior inferior cerebellar artery (PICA) territory infarctions may mimic labyrinthine disorders. A helpful distinction is that labyrinthine disease causes unidirectional nystagmus with fast component away from the side of the lesion and swaying toward the side of the lesion. In cerebellar infarction, the nystagmus is direction changing and more prominent toward the side of the lesion with swaying toward the side of the lesion.

REFERENCES

1. Bernat JL, Hunter RW: The benign lateral medullary syndrome. Arch Neurol 35:112, 1978.
2. Caplan LR: Vertebrobasilar disease: time for a new strategy. Curr Concepts Cerebrov Dis 15(3): July-Aug., 1980.
3. Caplan LR: The extracranial vertebral artery. Curr Concepts Cereb Dis 19(5):25, 1984.
4. Currier RD, Giles CL, DeJong RN: Some comments on Wallenberg's lateral medullary syndrome. Neurology 11:778, 1961.
5. Kistler JP, et al: Therapy of ischemic cerebral vascular disease due to atherosclerosis. N Engl J Med 311:27, 100, 1984.

EYE PAIN, LOSS OF VISION, AND EXOPHTHALMOS

<u>CASE 33</u>: A 29-year-old, married man presented with a 6-month history of slowly progressive "blurred" vision in his right eye and supraorbital pain. There were no other symptoms. Examination revealed right exophthalmos, acuity in the right eye of 20/50, and pallor of the right optic disc. There was papilledema on the left. The rest of the examination was normal. A skull X-ray revealed thickening of the bones of the right orbit and a CT scan revealed a right intraorbital and anterior temporal mass. A carotid arteriogram revealed supply of the mass from the right external and internal carotid arteries.

NEUROANATOMICAL CLUE: Label the numbered structures on this basal view of the skull, each of which is a known location for this type of tumor.

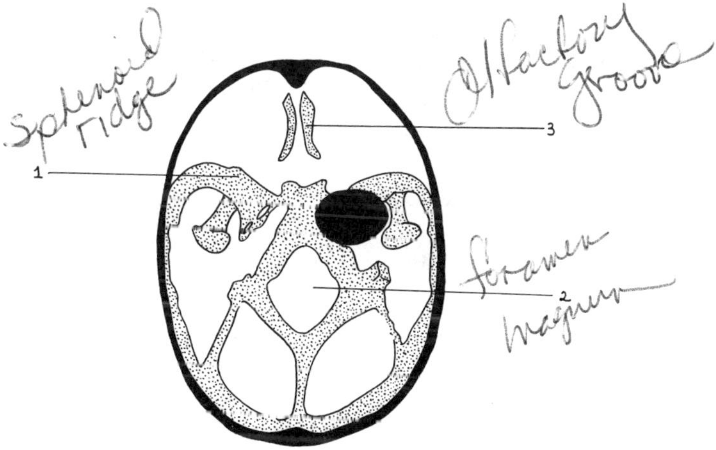

QUESTIONS:

1. What is the most likely diagnosis? What are the most common locations for this type of tumor?

2. How do these tumors usually present?

3. What is the recommended treatment?

4. Name the common histological types of this tumor.

5. What are the most helpful laboratory aids in diagnosis?

ANSWERS:

1. Sphenoid ridge meningioma. Parasagittal and falx (24%), convexity (18%), sphenoid ridge (18%), olfactory groove (10%), suprasellar (10%), posterior fossa (9%), other locations (11%).

   NEUROANATOMICAL CLUE:

   1 - Sphenoid ridge

   2 - Foramen magnum

   3 - Olfactory groove

2. It depends on the location, e.g., parasagittal meningiomas usually present with headache, personality change, and evidence of frontal lobe dysfunction; olfactory groove meningiomas often present with headache and visual loss - anosmia is nearly always present on exam.

3. Complete microsurgical removal is usually attempted; when this is not possible and/or when tumor is histologically malignant, or clinically invasive, radiotherapy may be useful.

4. Syncytial, transitional, fibroblastic, angioblastic, malignant. Tumors frequently show gradations among the various types.

5. Skull X-ray, CT scan, arteriogram.

PEARLS:

1. Convexity meningiomas commonly cause seizures.

2. Meningiomas, although usually benign, may occur in "malignant" locations (e.g., intraventricular).

3. A meningioma of the inner third of the sphenoid ridge may cause ipsilateral optic atrophy and contralateral papilledema (Foster Kennedy syndrome), as in this case.

4. A meningioma offers the prospect of cure with total extirpation.

5. Skull X-ray changes of hyperostosis and increased vascularity may be clues to an underlying meningioma.

PITFALLS:

1. Clivus meningiomas may be confused with intrinsic brainstem lesions.

2. Foramen magnum meningiomas, which account for 8% of posterior fossa meningiomas, may present with cervical pain and arm weakness/numbness and masquerade as cervical spondylosis. Young patients with foramen magnum meningioma may be incorrectly diagnosed as having multiple sclerosis.

3. Multiple meningiomas are seen in association with neurofibromatosis.

4. Recurrence of intracranial meningiomas after apparently complete surgical removal occurs in approximately 10% of patients.

REFERENCES

1. Chan RC, Thompson GB: Morbidity, mortality, and quality of life following surgery for intracranial meningiomas. A retrospective study in 257 cases. J Neurosurg 60:52, 1984.
2. Forbes AR, Goldberg ID: Radiation therapy in the treatment of meningioma: The Joint Center for Radiation Therapy experience 1970 to 1982. J Clin Oncol 2:1139, 1984.
3. Quest DO: Meningiomas: An update. Neurosurgery 3(2):219, 1978.
4. Rosenbaum AE: Meningiomas revisited. Semin Roentgenol 19(1):115, 1984.
5. Rosenberg LF, Miller NR: Visual results after microsurgical removal of meningiomas involving the anterior visual system. Arch Ophthalmol 102:1019, 1984.
6. Susac J, et al: The impossible meningioma. Arch Neurol 34:36, 1977.

ANALGESIA AND WEAKNESS OF THE HANDS IN A YOUNG WOMAN

CASE 34: A 31-year-old Mexican woman was evaluated because of weakness of her hands. Five years earlier she had sustained a burn of her right hand which was painless. Over the next 2 years she developed numbness, which began in her hands and later spread to her feet. Subsequently, the numbness spread to more proximal parts of her arms and legs. She was born and raised in an upper class neighborhood in Mexico and there was no family history of neurologic disease.

On examination, vital signs were normal and there was no orthostatic hypotension. Skin was remarkable for multiple traumatic scars on her hands. Cranial nerve examination revealed weakness of the muscles of eye closure (orbicularis oculi) and weakness of the medial, but not of the lateral, brow muscles (frontalis). In her extremities, muscle bulk was reduced and there was diffuse weakness which was more prominent distally than proximally; her hands were completely paralyzed and she could barely flex or extend her wrists against gravity. Deep tendon reflexes were within normal limits (2+/5) throughout and plantar responses were flexor. There was reduced pain and temperature perception below the elbows and knees. Position, vibration, and touch perception and cerebellar function and gait were normal.

QUESTIONS:

1. What is the significance of a "dissociated" sensory loss; i.e., the loss of pain/temperature sensation with preservation of position/vibration sensation?

2. What are the important causes of this type of sensory loss?

3. What further workup would you recommend?

4. Nerve conduction studies revealed decreased amplitudes of compound muscle action potentials and normal nerve conduction velocities. Electromyogram (EMG) revealed many fibrillation potentials in distal muscle groups. What is the significance of these results?

5. A sural nerve biopsy revealed perineural granulomas. What is the most likely diagnosis?

NEUROANATOMICAL CLUE: Weakness of the medial but not lateral aspect of the frontalis muscle is a classic symptom of this disease and the differential involvement of this muscle is explained by regional differences in forehead temperature.

ANSWERS:

1. Pain/temperature sensation may be lost independent of vibration/position sensation in _peripheral nerve_ disease and in _spinal cord_ disease. In peripheral nerve small, unmyelinated, and lightly myelinated fibers carry pain and temperature sensation, whereas large, thickly myelinated fibers carry position and vibration sensation. In the spinal cord, pain and temperature fibers, upon entering, decussate anterior to the central canal, whereas vibration and position fibers ascend in the spinal cord ipsilaterally without crossing.

2. _Syringomyelia_ is the classic spinal cord disease which produces a dissociated sensory loss (see case 25) by involving decussating pain and temperature fibers adjacent to the central canal. Because syrinxes usually occur in the cervical area, one would not expect to find a dissociated sensory loss in the lower extremities, as was the case with this patient. In terms of peripheral nerve disease, the classic diseases of small unmyelinated fibers are _amyloidosis_ and _leprosy_.

3. _Nerve conduction studies and nerve biopsy are indicated_. A myelogram to assess the width of the spinal cord (the spinal cord is widened in syringomyelia and in intramedullary tumors) was indicated if the correct diagnosis remained in doubt.

4. A decrease in the amplitude of nerve conduction action potentials occurs with primary axonal disease. A decrease in nerve conduction velocity occurs in diseases which produce Schwann cell injury and demyelination. These studies indicate that this patient's disease involves _axons_ primarily and that there is little, if any, demyelination present.

5. Granulomas imply chronic inflammation and are usually present with certain infections and foreign bodies. Perineural and epineural granulomas are most commonly seen in leprosy. In this case, staining for acid-fast organisms revealed numerous bacilli that were histologically typical of mycobacterium leprae (_leprosy_). It is very unusual for sarcoidosis or tuberculosis to involve nerve.

PEARLS:

1. In patients with peripheral neuropathy and brisk reflexes, think of amyloidosis and leprosy. These are the most important "small fiber" neuropathies.

2. The neuropathic manifestations of leprosy can vary from a single hypopigmented patch of cutaneous anesthesia (tuberculoid leprosy) to a severe disabling peripheral neuropathy (lepromatous leprosy).

3. The leprosy bacillus multiplies and spreads subcutaneously and has a predilection for cool areas of skin; this accounts for the characteristic facial distribution of anesthesia in the pinnae of the ears, tip of the nose, and medial aspects of the forehead.

4. Prominent autonomic symptoms (diarrhea, impotence, hypotension, etc.) are found in amyloidosis but are rare in leprosy.

5. In patients with proximal neuropathy ("bathing suit" distribution), think of porphyria.

6. Treatment of leprosy involves long-term therapy with sulfone medication, most commonly with Dapsone.

PITFALLS:

1. Leprosy is the most common cause of peripheral neuropathy in the world today. Think of leprosy in patients with unexplained peripheral neuropathy. Endemic foci are present in parts of the southern United States.

2. In patients with unexplained neuropathy, it is essential to examine as many family members as possible; in one recent study, 42% of patients referred because of unexplained neuropathy were found to have familial neuropathy.

REFERENCES

1. Case records of the Massachusetts General Hospital. N Engl J Med, p. 546, 1979 (this case was a formal presentation of the patient discussed in this case history).
2. Dyck PJ: Current Concepts in Neurology. The causes, classification, and treatment of peripheral neuropathy. N Engl J Med 307:283, 1982.
3. Dyck PJ, Oviatt KF, Lambert EH: Intensive evaluation of referred, unclassified neuropathies yields improved diagnosis. Ann Neurol 10:222, 1981.
4. Levis WR: Treatment of leprosy in the United States. Bull NY Acad Med 60:696, 1984.
5. Sabin TD: Temperature-linked sensory loss: a unique pattern in leprosy. Arch Neurol 20:257, 1969.
6. Sabin TD, Swift TR: Leprosy, In _Peripheral Neuropathy_, PJ Dyck, PK Thomas, and EH Lambert (Eds). Philadelphia, W.B. Saunders, p. 1166, 1975.

SEIZURES, COMA, AND ANEMIA

CASE 35: A 47-year-old woman was admitted in coma. One month earlier she had a generalized seizure, was found to be anemic, and was given a transfusion. She subsequently had been irritable and complained of headache. A second seizure prompted her admission. Physical examination found a comatose woman who responded only to painful stimuli. The disc margins were slightly blurred. There was generalized hyperreflexia and bilateral Babinski responses. A CT scan was normal. Hemoglobin, 9.8 gm%; hematocrit, 30%. Red blood cells appeared unusual (see below). A spinal tap revealed opening pressure of 280; closing pressure, 180; 854 red cells; 36 WBC; glucose, 75 mg%; protein 147 mg%; cultures all negative. After appropriate therapy, the patient made a full recovery.

QUESTIONS:

1. What is the connection between this patient's seizures, anemia, and high spinal fluid protein?

2. Name the two laboratory tests used to confirm the diagnosis.

3. Name the three agents useful in treating this disorder.

4. How can X-rays be helpful in diagnosis?

LABORATORY CLUE: Appearance of red blood cells in this case:

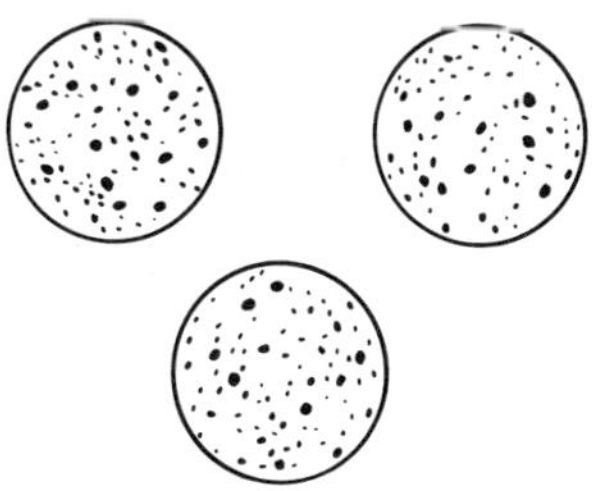

ANSWERS:

1. *Lead poisoning*, which in this case was due to high lead content in this patient's home drinking water. The toxic effects of lead are related to increases in its concentration in the soft tissues of the body.

2. Blood lead level; free erythrocyte protoporphyrin (FEP) level.

3. Calcium disodium edetate (CaNa EDTA); dimercaprol; penicillamine.

4. *Lead lines* at metaphyses of long bones may be visible; negative X-rays do *not* rule out lead poisoning.

LABORATORY CLUE: Basophilic stippling in red blood cells in lead intoxication.

PEARLS:

1. a) Seizures, anemia, high cerebrospinal fluid protein: Think of lead poisoning.

   b) Irritability, clumsiness, and abdominal pain in a child: Think of lead poisoning.

2. The most common sources of exposure to lead are ingestion of paint or of fluids stored in lead pipes or tanks; inhalation of automobile emissions or of dust containing lead in lead related industries.

3. *Chronic heavy metal exposure* usually causes headache, drowsiness, confusion, and peripheral neuropathy.

4. Appropriate *supportive therapy* is as vital to survival as chelating agents in the treatment of lead intoxication. Measures include careful attention to fluid and electrolytes, and control of seizures.

4. Common heavy metal toxicity that may occur in industry includes lead, arsenic, manganese, and mercury.

PITFALLS:

1. A *spinal tap may be dangerous* in lead intoxication due to increased intracranial pressure. In this case, the correct diagnosis was not suspected until after the lumbar puncture was performed.

2. Temporary exacerbation of lead encephalopathy may occur in the early stages of treatment with chelating agents.

3. "Asymptomatic" patients with elevated body lead levels may have subtle problems with intellectual function, and behavioral abnormalities.

REFERENCES

1. Charney E, Kessler B, Farfel M, Jackson D: Childhood lead poisoning. A controlled trial of the effect of dust-control measures on blood lead levels. N Engl J Med 309:1089, 1983.
2. Chisolm JL, Barltrop D: Recognition and management of children with increased lead absorption. Arch Dis Child 54:249, 1979.
3. Keogh JP: Recognizing lead poisoning in adults. Arch Int Med 144:1944, 1984.
4. King E: Lead poisoning. Pub Health Rev 10:49, 1982.
5. Pincus D, Saccar C: Lead poisoning. Am Fam Physician 19:120, 1979.
6. Piomelli S, Rosen JF, Chisolm JJ Jr, Graef JW: Management of childhood lead poisoning. J Pediatr 105:523, 1984.

LEFT HEMIPLEGIA IN AN AIRLINE PILOT

CASE 36: A 45-year-old, right-handed commercial airline pilot was brought into the emergency room by his copilot because of a left hemiplegia. The previous day he successfully piloted a cross-country flight but, after landing, appeared uncharacteristically garrulous, loud, and inappropriate. He required help to get to his hotel room and, in retrospect, appeared to have been confused. The following morning he was found on the floor at the foot of his bed unable to move his left side.

Examination revealed a robust appearing man with a left hemiplegia. Vital signs were normal. He was alert, speech was normal, and he was fully oriented. He was not totally aware of his deficits and occasionally made inappropriate jokes. When asked what was wrong, he responded "Nothing. I just came in for a checkup." When asked why he was not moving his left side, he responded that it had "just fallen asleep for several minutes."

Examination showed a complete left hemiplegia equally involving face, arm, and leg and marked inattention to the left side of the body. At rest, eyes were deviated to the right. There appeared to be sensory deficits on the left to pinch, touch, and to vibration, although examination was difficult because of neglect of that side. Reflexes were decreased on the left and the left plantar response was extensor. General examination was unremarkable and, in particular, the patient was afebrile and there was no organomegaly, cardiac murmur, or carotid bruit present.

QUESTIONS:

1. What area of the nervous system was involved? What are the characteristic symptoms when this area of the CNS is involved?

2. Laboratory studies showed: CBC - normochromic, normocytic anemia, normal white blood count and platelet count; sedimentation rate - 120 mm per hour; elevated alkaline phosphatase, SGOT, and LDH levels. How might these abnormalities relate to this patient's acute neurologic illness?

3. An ECHO cardiogram and lumbar puncture were normal. CT scan revealed a decrease in the size of the right lateral ventricle compatible with early swelling of the right hemisphere; there was no contrast enhancement. A right carotid arteriogram showed occlusion of the right internal carotid artery. Could this be herpes encephalitic?

4. What are important causes of stroke in young patients to be considered?

5. What workup would you now recommend?

ANSWERS:

1. Nondominant parietal lobe lesions produce anosognosia (loss of awareness of deficits), inattention, abnormalities in spatial orientation, dressing apraxia, and constructional apraxia (difficulty copying geometric figures).

2. Elevated sedimentation rates are characteristically seen in patients with a) infection, b) malignancy, and c) chronic inflammatory and autoimmune diseases. The normochromic-normocytic anemia is consistent with a chronic disease and abnormalities of liver function tests also suggest systemic disease in this patient.

3. The CT scan is consistent with an early right hemisphere infarction. An acute infectious illness of the brain, such as herpes simplex encephalitis, is unlikely without fever, with a normal CSF profile, and in the absence of CT enhancement. The arteriogram was consistent with a large embolic occlusion of the right internal carotid artery.

4. a) Cardiac lesions, including rheumatic valve disease, mitral valve prolapse, and paradoxical embolus through a patent foramen ovale; b) carotid dissection, spontaneous or traumatic; c) hypercoagulable states associated with malignancy, chronic inflammatory diseases (e.g., lupus erythematosus), or hematologic diseases (polycythemia and thrombocytosis); d) in women, pregnancy and birth control use in susceptible individuals; e) drug use, especially cocaine and amphetamines, predisposes to intracerebral vasculitis and stroke.

5. A complete medical evaluation is indicated to determine the source of the elevated sedimentation rate, anemia, and abnormal liver function tests. Chest X-ray in this patient disclosed multiple parenchymal blastic and lytic bony lesions, and he was subsequently found to have widely metastatic carcinoma of the prostate. The stroke probably resulted from a hypercoagulable state secondary to his primary illness and may have been due to nonbacterial thrombotic endocarditis, which is an important cause of embolic stroke in patients with disseminated cancer.

PEARLS:

1. In patients with acute stroke, always look for other evidence of arterial embolization. Emboli to the extremities may result in a pale, cool limb, renal emboli may produce hematuria, and emboli to the bowel usually cause abdominal pain.

2. With <u>cortical</u> lesions, eyes deviate <u>away</u> from the hemiparesis; with <u>brainstem</u> lesions, eyes deviate <u>toward</u> the hemiparesis.

3. CT scans performed within 24 hours of an acute stroke may be normal; a normal CT scan does not rule out a thrombotic or embolic cerebrovascular accident. CT scans 2-3 days following a thrombotic or embolic stroke are usually abnormal but may show contrast enhancement and be mistaken for a brain tumor. CT scans in patients with intracerebral hemorrhage are invariably positive immediately.

4. Patients with systemic lupus erythematosus may have brain emboli due to noninfectious endocarditis (Libman-Sacks endocarditis).

PITFALLS:

1. Confusion or a change in behavior may be the major symptom of a <u>nondominant hemisphere stroke</u> and the diagnosis is frequently missed in these patients.

2. Rehabilitation of patients with nondominant strokes is often unsuccessful because of persistent anosognosia (failure to recognize deficits) and poor motivation.

REFERENCES

1. Barnett HJM, et al. Further evidence relating mitral-valve prolapse to cerebral ischemic events. N Engl J Med 302:139, 1980.
2. Barron KD, Siquera E, Hirano A. Cerebral embolism caused by non-bacterial thrombotic endocarditis. Neurology 10:39, 1960.
3. Easton D, Sherman P: Management of cerebral embolism of cardiac origin. Stroke 11:433, 1980.
4. Graus F, Rogers LR, Posner JB: Cerebrovascular complications in patients with cancer. Medicine 64:16, 1985.
5. Kooklier JC: Cerebral embolism, marantic endocarditis, and cancer. Arch Neurol 33(4):260, 1976.
6. Posner JB: Neurologic complications of systemic cancer. Disease a Month. Chicago, Year Book Publishers 25(2) Nov. 1978.
7. Rosen P, Armstrong D: Non-bacterial thrombotic endocarditis in patients with malignant neoplastic diseases. Am J Med 54:23, 1973.

A YOUNG WOMAN WITH FALLING SPELLS

CASE 37: A 23-year-old mother of two was self-referred for evaluation of falling spells. She had spent her entire life in a rural area of northern Maine. At age 16, shortly after the birth of her first child, she developed frequent falling spells. Typically, she would suddenly lose all motor control, fall to the ground, and remain unable to move or to even cry out for help. These episodes would typically last for several seconds and, although they sometimes appeared to occur spontaneously, they often were precipitated by anger or laughter. She reported that whenever she screamed at one of her children, she would suddenly fall mute and helpless. At no time did she lose consciousness. These spells occurred as often as 15 times daily and resulted in a 4-year hospitalization in a local psychiatric inpatient facility. Intensive psychiatric care failed to reveal the source of these episodes or to lessen their frequency.

She also reported daytime episodes of intense sleepiness followed by brief periods of sleep, after which she would awaken refreshed. These episodes occurred approximately monthly and occasionally would begin while she was standing talking to people. As an adolescent, she also experienced "nightmares while I was falling asleep," consisting of terrifying visual hallucinations.

General physical and neurological evaluation was notable only for mild obesity. Family history was negative for neuropsychiatric disease.

QUESTIONS:

1. What is the most likely explanation for this woman's falling spells? What other diseases should be considered?

2. What associated symptoms may occur with this disease?

3. What is the etiology of this disorder?

4. How are patients with these symptoms best treated?

ANSWERS:

1. Cataplexy which consists of sudden loss of muscle tone, usually induced by an emotional response, such as laughter, crying, or anger. Attacks of cataplexy are very brief, lasting only seconds, and are never associated with loss of consciousness. The differential diagnosis includes seizure disorders, particularly akinetic seizures and partial complex (temporal lobe) seizures. Patients with hypokalemic and normokalemic periodic paralysis do not lose and regain motor control as rapidly as did this patient.

2. Cataplexy most often occurs, as it did in this patient, in association with narcolepsy. Patients may also experience sleep paralysis, consisting of paralysis during the transition between wakefulness and sleep, and hypnagogic hallucinations, consisting of intense visual or auditory experiences while falling asleep or awakening. These four symptoms together form the narcolepsy tetrad.

3. Narcolepsy represents a biological disorder of the sleep-wake cycle. There is no evidence that narcolepsy is psychosomatic or psychological in origin. In patients with narcolepsy and cataplexy, attacks of sleep are associated with sudden changes in the electroencephalogram (EEG) from normal to REM sleep.

4. Narcolepsy is best treated by dextroamphetamine sulfate (Dexedrine), by methylphenidate hydrochloride (Ritalin), or pemoline (Cylert). These drugs decrease REM sleep. Narcolepsy and hyperactive behavior disorders in children are the only indications for amphetamine treatment in neurologic medicine. Cataplexy is best treated with tricyclic antidepressants, such as Imipramine or protriptyline. This patient responded to Imipramine with a complete disappearance of her falling spells.

PEARLS:

1. Narcolepsy usually begins between adolescence and age 30 and occurs more frequently after meals and late in the day. Episodes of uncontrollable sleep are generally short-lived, lasting less than 15 minutes, and the patient awakens refreshed.

2. Occasionally, patients with narcolepsy are effectively treated by planning <u>short naps</u> periodically during the day.

3. Patients with <u>craniopharyngioma</u> or other disorders of the hypothalamus may have narcolepsy-like symptoms. The possibility that narcolepsy may be secondary to another CNS disease should be considered in all patients.

4. The Kleine-Levin syndrome consists of episodic hypersomnia and bulimia (overeating) and occurs almost exclusively in obese males.

5. Sleep centers have been established in a number of university hospitals for the study and treatment of patients with refractory sleep disorders. Continuous EEG monitoring of patients while asleep can help establish the correct diagnosis and suggest the appropriate therapy.

PITFALLS:

1. In patients with cataplexy-like symptoms who do not have associated narcolepsy, the careful exclusion of epilepsy is important.

2. <u>Narcolepsy is not a rare disease</u>. The estimated incidence is 0.07% in the United States. The most common cause of hypersomnia in the United States is depression.

3. Patients with cataplexy may sustain serious falls and injuries.

4. Other important causes of <u>chronic fatigue</u> and <u>sleepiness</u> include: hypothyroidism, drug use and abuse, morbid obesity, and chronic medical illnesses.

REFERENCES

1. Guilleminault C, Dement WC: 235 cases of excessive daytime sleepiness: diagnosis and tentative classification. J Neurol Psychiatry 31:13, 1977.
2. Guilleminault C, Dement WC, Passouant P (Eds): Narcolepsy, New York, Spectrum 1976.
3. Kales A, Cadieux RJ, PolDatos CR, et al: Narcolepsy-cataplexy. I. Clinical and electrophysiological characteristics. II. Psychosocial consequences and associated psychopathology. Arch Neurol 39:164, 1982.
4. Kales A, Kales JD: Sleep disorders. Recent findings in the diagnosis and treatment of disturbed sleep. N Engl J Med 290:487, 1974.
5. Richardson GF: Excessive daytime sleepiness in man: Multiple sleep latency measurement in narcoleptic and control subjects. Electroencephalogr Clin Neurophysiol 425:621, 1978.
6. Roth T, et al: Sleepiness: its measurement and determinants. Sleep 5(Suppl 2):128, 1982.
7. Zarcone V: Narcolepsy. N Engl J Med 288:1156, 1973.

AMNESIA IN A MIDDLE-AGED MAN

CASE 38: A 57-year-old bus driver was brought in by his family because of an acute confusional state. They reported that during dinner he appeared perfectly normal, but that within minutes of getting up from the table he suddenly appeared startled and confused and began running back and forth between his wife and children, grabbing them and shouting repeatedly "What's all this?" They brought him immediately to the emergency room.

His medical history was remarkable for hypertension of 5 years' duration which had been well controlled with diuretics. He was on no other medications, was not known to abuse alcohol, and had no prior history of abnormal behavior.

On examination, he was an obese man, who appeared excited and afraid. He repeatedly grabbed the examiner at the shoulders with both hands and asked "What's all this?" or "What's going on?" When reassured, he would relax momentarily, but then become agitated again. His speech was normal and he could introduce himself and the members of his family appropriately. He did not know the date or year and was unable to supply any details of his current illness or of the ride to the hospital. He incorrectly reported that he was working for a bus company whose employ he had actually left 2 years ago. When reminded of this by his wife, the patient had no recollection of leaving that previous job or of beginning a new job. Memories of the distant past, i.e., greater than 5 years ago, were normal. However, he was unable to recall any events which occurred within the past 2 years. Immediate recall of a series of 7 numbers presented to the patient was normal, but he was unable to recall any of 5 objects at 5 minutes. The remainder of a detailed neurologic and physical examination was normal.

QUESTIONS:

1. What are the 3 different types of memory? What type of memory loss did this patient have?

2. What type of memory disorder occurs following trauma? With seizures? With chronic alcohol abuse?

3. Why is this patient unlikely to have suffered a stroke?

4. What is the most likely explanation for this patient's illness?

5. What is the prognosis? What treatment should be given?

ANSWERS:

1. a) Immediate memory - ability to repeat information presented moments before; lost only in severe dementia and in inattentive/delirious states. b) Intermediate memory - "limbic" memory - temporal cortex and Papez circuit. c) Remote memory - diffuse cortical storage. This patient had a loss of intermediate memory.

2. a) Following trauma, a loss of intermediate or "limbic" memory may occur with an inability to make new memories (anterograde memory loss). With recovery, the duration of retrograde memory loss decreases. b) With psychomotor (temporal lobe) seizures patients may appear to be amnestic, but they are also unable to carry out complex commands. c) Alcohol abuse may produce a "limbic" memory loss with confabulation and apathy (Korsakoff's syndrome); acutely, this may be associated with ataxia, quiet confusion, and disordered eye movements (Wernicke-Korsakoff syndrome). The acute disorder is due to thiamine deficiency and is usually reversible.

3. Memory loss without signs of focal neurologic disease is unlikely to be due to a stroke.

4. Transient global amnesia. Etiology not known, but most likely due to ischemia of the temporal lobes. This disorder is usually seen in middle-aged individuals with hypertension or with other risk factors for vascular disease. Many attacks are preceded by an emotionally charged event. It is of note that a single artery appears to supply both medial temporal lobes (Percheron's artery).

5. The prognosis for complete recovery within 12-48 hours is excellent. No special treatment need be given, except to treat the risk factor for stroke if present (e.g., hypertension, hypercholesterolemia). Some physicians put these patients on aspirin. Recurrent episodes of transient global amnesia occur in a minority of patients (10-20%), and in this group anticoagulation may be reasonable.

PEARLS:

1. Amnesia occurs with bilateral temporal lobe disease; subtle deficits may be present with lesions of the dominant temporal lobe.

2. A chronic loss of memory may occur in patients with cancer, usually oat-cell carcinoma of the lung or Hodgkin's disease. This disorder, of unknown cause, is referred to as "limbic encephalitis".

3. Ex-boxers may develop amnesia associated with abnormalities in speech and gait, and with associated extrapyramidal features ("dementia pugilistica" or "the punch-drunk syndrome"). This syndrome is thought to result from the effects of repeated small injuries.

4. Acute herpes simplex virus encephalitis typically affects the medial temporal lobes, but is unlikely to cause amnesia without associated findings, such as fever, seizures, stupor, aphasia, or hemiplegia.

5. An isolated inability to recognize faces, termed prosopagnosia, occurs with bilateral disease of the occipital-temporal lobe connections. These patients always have associated visual field abnormalities (hemianopsia or quadrantanopsia). Prosopagnosia is usually due to posterior cerebal artery vascular disease.

PITFALLS

1. Acute memory loss can result from a stroke in the territory of the posterior cerebral arteries. Careful examination for other symptoms of posterior circulation stroke (e.g., visual field defects) is essential in all patients with acute memory loss.

2. The patient who arrives at the hospital claiming not to remember who he is is likely hysterical or malingering. This type of memory loss, popularized in early Hollywood films, does not occur with known neurologic disease.

3. Patients who complain of memory loss are often depressed rather than amnesic. In true amnesia, patients are usually unable to recall their inability to recall.

REFERENCES

1. Casson IR, Siegel O, Sham R, Campbell EA, Tarlau M, DiDomenico A: Brain damage in modern boxers. JAMA 251:2663, 1984.
2. Corsellis JAN, Goldberg GJ, Norton AR: Limbic encephalitis and its association with carcinoma. Brain 91:481, 1968.
3. Crowell GF, Stump DA, et al: The transient global amnesia-migraine connection. Arch Neurol 41:75, 1984.
4. Fisher CM: Transient global amnesia: precipitating activities and other observations. Arch Neurol 39:605, 1982.
5. Fisher CM, Adams RD: Transient global amnesia. Acta Neurol Scand 40(Suppl 9):47, 1964.
6. Lampert PW, Hardman JM: Morphologic changes in brains of boxers. JAMA 251:2676, 1984.
7. Logan W, Sherman DG: Transient global amnesia. Curr Concepts Cerebrovasc Dis 18(3):May-June 1983.
8. Mathew NT, Meyer JS: Pathogenesis and natural history of transient global amnesia. Stroke 5:303, 1974.
9. Nausieda PA, Sherman IC: Long-term prognosis in transient global amnesia. JAMA 241:392, 1979.
10. Shiping JR, et al: Transient global amnesia. Ann Neurol 7:281, 1980.

THREE YOUNG MEN WITH ACUTE NEUROLOGIC SIGNS

CASE 39:

A) A 31-year-old recently married lawyer developed a sudden right hemiplegia while having breakfast with his partner. He was a successful amateur squash player and during the past week had been competing daily in a local tournament. One day earlier, he had complained to his wife of some left-sided neck pain and wondered whether he had strained a muscle in the tournament.

On examination, he was awake but mute and was totally without comprehension of spoken or written language. Eyes were deviated to the left. There was a dense right hemiplegia involving face, arm, and leg and an associated hemianesthesia. Reflexes were decreased on the right and the right plantar response was extensor. Palpation of facial pulses revealed reversal of flow of the left supraorbital pulse suggesting an internal carotid artery occlusion.

B) A 28-year-old manager of a convenience food market was admitted because of a transient episode of right arm numbness and weakness. One day earlier, there was an attempted robbery at his store which was discovered by local police, and for a 3-hour period he was held hostage at knife-point while the police and criminals negogiated his release. During this time, his arms were tied behind him and a knife was held tightly against his throat. He was released without harm. That evening, while at home and reading the newspaper, he noticed the sudden onset of numbness in right hand ("as if my hand fell asleep") and an inability to hold the paper with his right hand. That episode lasted 3-4 minutes and then resolved completely. He came in for evaluation at the insistence of his wife. Examination was within normal limits.

C) A 42-year-old fireman developed dizziness and diplopia while at work. It happened suddenly while he was high on a ladder fighting a poorly controlled fire in a chemical plant. He recalled that noxious smoke and heat was pouring out of the windows and he had to keep stretching his body and neck away from the building to avoid the fumes and to obtain breathable air. He suddenly felt vertiginous and had to be helped down by his colleagues. The vertigo persisted and his gait was noted to be unstable.

On arrival in the emergency room, he was alert and vital signs were normal. Speech was normal. He had frequent hiccups. Examination of eye movements showed horizontal nystagmus most marked on right gaze with the fast component to the right. There was a right hemiataxia involving both arm and leg. Neurologic examination was otherwise normal. CT scans obtained at admission were normal in each above case.

QUESTIONS:

1. What area of the CNS was affected in patient A? patient B? patient C?

2. Arteriograms demonstrated the same underlying pathologic finding in each patient. An example is given below. What is the finding?

3. What is the most likely explanation to account for this finding in each patient?

4. How would you treat patient A? patient B? patient C?

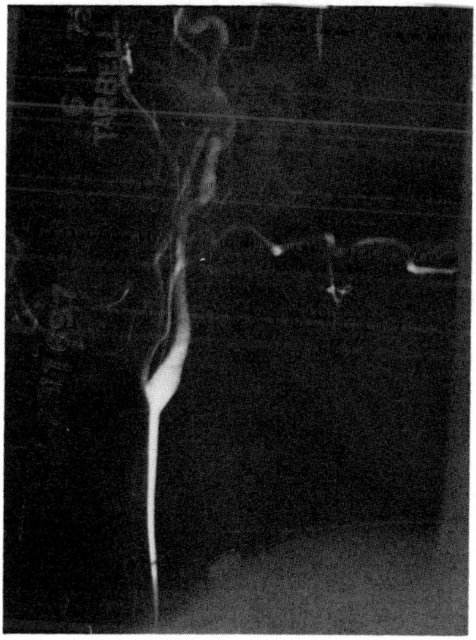

ANSWERS:

1. Patient A - extensive involvement of left hemisphere, probably frontal and parietal lobes, in vascular distribution of middle cerebral artery. Patient B - left hemisphere, focal involvement in area of prefrontal and postfrontal gyrus consistent with distribution of branches of the superior division, middle cerebral artery. Patient C - right posterior and lateral medulla, area of vestibular nuclei and inferior cerebellar peduncle, in distribution of vertebral artery.

2. Arterial dissections were found in each patient. In case A, a large dissection of the left internal carotid artery with complete obstruction of flow distally was present. In case B, a dissection with partial obstruction was found in the same vessel. In case C, a right vertebral artery dissection with partial obstruction was found.

3. In each case, the dissection was most likely the result of an injury to the vessel wall incurred during stretching of the neck or to direct trauma.

4. Patient A has suffered a massive, complete infarction in the territory of a major vessel and is unlikely to benefit from therapy. Patient B was treated for a transient ischemic attack with a 6 month course of anticoagulation. Patient C sustained an incomplete infarction within a vascular territory and was also treated with anticoagulation for a 6-month period. A follow-up arteriogram in case C 6 months later revealed a complete disappearance of the dissection.

PEARLS:

1. Many "spontaneous" dissections occur in patients with atherosclerosis and follow hemorrhage into a subintimal plaque.

2. There is an increased incidence of aortic and carotid dissections in patients with Marfan's syndrome.

3. Carotidynia, or pain along the course of the carotid artery in the neck, may take the form of recurrent attacks in young people or may occur in association with migraine.

4. Carotid dissections may be completely asymptomatic or may result in massive strokes. The dissection itself may be asymptomatic and neurologic symptoms may follow weeks or months later due to emboli from a clot forming at the site of the dissection.

5. Long, thin, distal segments of the internal carotid artery in dissections give the "string sign" appearance.

PITFALLS:

1. Do not massage carotid arteries, particularly in elderly patients.

2. Carotidynia may be a benign manifestation of migraine or may be a prelude to carotid occlusion.

REFERENCES

1. Fisher CM: The headache and pain of spontaneous carotid dissection. Headache 20:60, 1982.
2. Fisher CM, Ojemann RG, Roberson GH: Spontaneous dissection of cervico-cerebral arteries. Can J Neurol Sci 5:9, 1978.
3. Gee W, Kaupp H, et al.: Spontaneous dissection of internal carotid arteries. Arch Surg 115:944, 1980.
4. Katirji MB, Reinmuth OM, Latchaw RE: Stroke due to vertebral artery injury. Arch Neurol 42:242, 1985.
5. Mokri B, Sundt T, Houser W: Spontaneous internal carotid dissection, hemicrania, and Horner's syndrome. Arch Neurol 36:677, 1979.
6. Ojemann RG, Fisher CM, Rich JC: Spontaneous dissecting aneurysm of the internal carotid artery. Stroke 3:434, 1972.
7. Rashin N, Prusiner S: Carotidynia. Neurology 27:43, 1977.

OLD HOMONYMOUS HEMIANOPSIA AND NEW HEADACHE

CASE 40: A 46-year-old internist was found at the age of 21 to have a left homonymous hemianopsia. A right carotid angiogram was normal. He was well until 7 days previously when, after swimming 15 minutes, he felt weak, light-headed, and nauseated. These symptoms resolved in 2 minutes. Three days later, again while swimming, he developed a sudden, excruciating, occipital headache radiating frontally and associated with dizziness, blurred vision, paresthesias in both hands and feet, nausea, and weakness. He told doctors in an outlying hospital that he thought he had had a subarachnoid hemorrhage. Examination at that time revealed a blood pressure of 130 mm Hg systolic, a slightly asymmetric smile, and a left knee jerk which was more brisk than the right. There was "twitching" of the right hand. The cerebrospinal fluid was xanthochromic and under a pressure of 550 mm H O. Later on the day of admission the paresthesias disappeared and by the following day the blurred vision cleared. He was then transferred to your hospital.

General examination was within normal limits. The neurologic examination, except for the left homonymous hemianopsia, was normal.

A CT scan and arteriogram were performed and appear on the opposite page.

QUESTIONS:

1. Describe the radiographic findings.

2. What are the most common presenting symptoms of this disease?

3. What familial syndromes are associated with this abnormality?

4. What is the natural history of this condition if untreated?

5. What treatment would you recommend?

NEUROANATOMICAL CLUE:

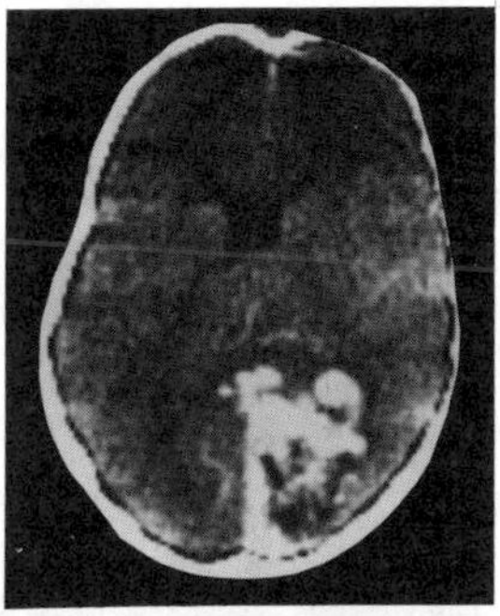

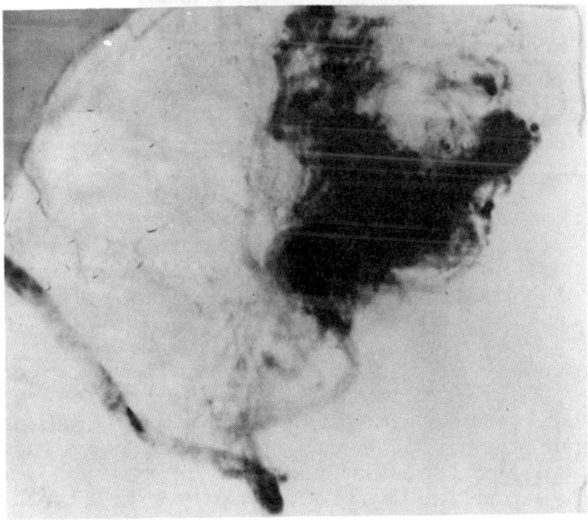

ANSWERS

1. The CT scan shows an area of contrast enhancement in the right occipial lobe with a typical pattern of an arteriovenous malformation (AVM); there is an adjacent low absorption area, presumably representing infarcted tissue. Arteriography demonstrates that the major arterial feeders of the arteriovenous malformation are from the right posterior cerebral artery. Other radiologic findings of arteriovenous malformation include calcifications which may appear as crescentic on skull X-rays.

2. AVMs can present for the first time as subarachnoid hemorrhage or as intracerebral hemorrhage (50% of patients), as focal or generalized seizures (35%), or may be discovered during a workup for chronic headache or for unexplained focal neurologic signs, such as hemiparesis.

3. a) Sturge-Weber disease - Port wine facial nevus and ipsilateral angioma. b) von Hippel-Lindau disease - retinal hemangioma and hemangioblastoma of cerebellum, brainstem or spinal cord; may have associated polycystic disease of kidney and pancreas. c) Klippel-Trenaunay syndrome - cutaneous vascular nevus and spinal cord vascular malformation. d) Osler-Weber-Rendu disease - AVMs of many organs, including central nervous system.

4. The natural history of untreated AVMs is incompletely known. It is likely that patients who have a history of a previous bleed, as did this patient, have a higher incidence of future bleeds, estimated at 4% per year for life.

5. Fifty percent of cerebral AVMs can be surgically removed. Surgical morbidity and mortality will depend upon the location and size of the malformation and on the experience of the surgeon. Most neurologists recommend surgical extirpation, if possible, of AVMs that have previously bled. Removal is also often recommended for AVMs that have not bled but are symptomatic and in surgically accessible locations. Alternative therapies include embolization, balloon ligation of feeding vessels, and low-dose proton beam therapy; none of these treatments have been subject to rigorous trials of efficacy.

PEARLS:

1. Headaches/seizures/intellectual deterioration - think of AVM.

2. In a young adult, a systolic bruit in the neck or over the eye or cranium is highly suggestive of an AVM. Exercise may amplify the bruit in some patients.

3. AVMs are congenital malformations of the nervous system. The vessels within these malformations tend to bleed because they have abnormally thin walls.

4. The syndrome of Foix-Alajouanine, consisting of progressive myelopathy of the thoracic cord and seen generally in middle-aged men, is due to an AVM of the spinal cord.

5. In most cases, the brain tissue within an AVM is not functioning properly and complete removal of the AVM usually will not result in an added neurological deficit. This is particularly true in children.

PITFALLS:

1. Slowly progressive neurologic deficits in patients with large AVMs are due to shunting of blood away from normal brain to the AVM ("steal") or to pressure effects from engorged vessels within the malformation.

2. Think of the possibility of venous malformations in patients with unexplained neurologic symptoms and with vascular nevi or other discolored areas of skin on the head, neck, or back.

3. Diagnosis of AVM is particularly difficult in the brainstem and spinal cord and may be mistaken for demyelinating disease.

4. Prior to consideration of surgery or other treatment, it is essential to define the exact distribution of the arterial feeders and venous drainage of an AVM.

REFERENCES

1. Berstrand A, Hook O, Lindvall H: Vascular malformations of spinal cord. Acta Neurol Scand 40:169, 1964.
2. Logue V: Angiomas of the spinal cord: Review of the pathogenesis, clinical features, and results of surgery. J Neurol Neurosurg Psychiatry 42:1, 1979.
3. Olivecrona H, Rieves J: Arteriovenous aneurysms of the brain: their diagnosis and treatment. Arch Neurol Psychiatry 59:567, 1948.
4. Parkinson D, Bachers G: Arteriovenous malformations. Summary of 100 consecutive supratentorial cases. J Neurosurg 53:285, 1980.
5. Poole JL: Treatment of arteriovenous malformations in the cerebral hemisphere. J Neurosurg 19:136, 1962.
6. Roman G, Fisher M, Perl DP, Poser CM: Neurological manifestations of hereditary hemorrhagic telangiectasia (Rendu-Osler-Weber Disease): Report of 2 cases and review of the literature. Ann Neurol 4:130, 1978.
7. Sampson D, Ditmore QM, Beyer CW Jr: Intravascular use of isobutyl 2-cyanoacrylate: I. Treatment of intracranial arteriovenous malformations. Neurosurgery 8:43, 1981.
8. Steiger HJ, Tew JM: Hemorrhage and epilepsy in cryptic cerebrovascular malformations. Arch Neurol 41:722, 1984.
9. Stein BM, Wolpert SM. Arteriovenous malformations of the brain: Current concepts of treatment. I and II. Arch Neurol 37:1-5, 69, 1980.
10. Wilson CB, U HS, Domenigue J: Microsurgical treatment of intracranial vascular malformations. J Neurosurg 51:446, 1979.

FEVER AND SHOCK IN AN ELDERLY WOMAN

CASE 41: A 67-year-old woman was brought into the emergency room by a friend because of fever and headache. For 36 hours she had complained of cough and joint pains.

Examination revealed a pleasant, bright woman, who appeared pale and in moderate pain. Blood pressure was 150/90. Pulse 96 and regular. Temperature 102.3 F. Examination of skin revealed several purpuric lesions on the abdomen and flank. There was resistance to neck flexion. At this point in the examination the patient suddenly lost consciousness. Recheck of vital signs revealed blood pressure of 40 systolic and pulse 140 and thready.

QUESTIONS:

1. What is the most likely cause of this patient's illness?

2. How should she be treated?

ANSWERS:

1. This is the classic picture of meningitis with *meningococcemia* and sudden circulatory collapse.

2. Immediate treatment is essential for *shock* (intravenous fluids, intravenous steroids, and, if necessary, pressors) and immediate treatment for meningococcemia with *penicillin G*, 12-24 million units per day. As the penicillin solution is prepared, blood cultures and lumbar puncture should be done. The lumbar puncture should not delay, and can be done simultaneously with the institution of therapy.

Follow-up: Lumbar puncture in this patient revealed an opening pressure of 400 mm H 0, cloudy fluid and a white count of 6,250/mm , 100% of CSF cells were polymorphonuclear leukocytes. CSF glucose was 0 mg% and CSF protein 245 mg%. With appropriate treatment, systolic blood pressure remained between 80 and 100 mm/mercury for 6 hours and then began to rise to normal levels. Twelve hours later, the patient was afebrile, awake, alert, and eating breakfast.

QUESTIONS:

1. Name the three most important causes of meningitis in adults?

2. What is the usual reservoir of meningococcus?

3. Should household contacts of this patient be treated?

4. What groups of patients are most susceptible to pneumococcal meningitis?

5. What are some important causes of recurrent meningitis?

ANSWERS:

1. Streptococcus (pneumococcus) 30-50%; Neisseria meningitidis (meningococcus) 10-30%; hemophilus influenza 1-3%.

2. Between epidemics, approximately 10% of healthy individuals harbor meningococcus in the nasopharynx; this percentage increases during epidemics and among contacts of patients with meningococcal meningitis. Infection with this organism can occur sporadically or as part of epidemics and military recruits have been particularly susceptible to infection. Meningococcus is the most important cause of epidemic bacterial meningitis.

3. Intimate household contacts of patients with meningococcemia should receive a 2-day course of rifampicin (600 mg per day). Alternatively, if infection is with group A or group C meningococcus, vaccines for household contacts are now available.

4. Think of pneumococcus as a cause of meningitis in patients with pneumonia or otitis media and in patients with alcoholism, sickle cell anemia, splenectomy, and basal skull fracture.

5. Fistulas are usually due to congenital neurectodermal sinuses, trauma (especially basilar skull fractures), and postsurgery. Mollaret's meningitis is a syndrome of recurrent meningitis of unknown cause.

PEARLS:

1. Blood cultures are critical in the evaluation of meningitis. Positive blood cultures are found in 50% of patients with meningitis and in some patients with negative CSF cultures.

2. Counterimmunoelectrophoresis can detect bacterial antigens in the CSF and is particularly useful in the diagnosis of partially treated bacterial meningitis.

3. In elderly, debilitated, or immunosuppressed patients, think of listeria monocytogenes and gram negative organisms as causes of bacterial meningitis.

4. In patients with bacterial meningitis due to anaerobes, think of <u>brain abscess</u> as the underlying etiology.

5. In most patients with meningitis therapy should be continued for 10-14 days. If the patient is doing well clinically, there is no need for repeat spinal taps.

PITFALLS:

1. <u>Stiff neck disappears</u> in the stuporous or comatose patient with meningitis.

2. During the first few hours of bacterial meningitis the <u>CSF may be completely acellular</u>, although bacteria may be visible on gram stain.

3. Suspicion of meningitis is an indication for <u>immediate lumbar puncture</u> in all circumstances. Do not delay lumbar puncture pending CT scan or other diagnostic procedures.

4. It is particularly important to <u>think</u> of meningitis in elderly and in alcoholic patients admitted because of confusion whether or not there is fever present.

5. Serum electrolytes should be followed carefully in patients with meningitis because of the potential complication of <u>inappropriate ADH secretion</u>.

REFERENCES

1. Beaty HN: Meningococcal infections. In <u>Harrison's Principles of Internal Medicine</u>, Petersdorf, et al. (Eds), 10th edition. New York, McGraw-Hill, pp. 935, 1983.
2. Fong W, Ranalli P: Staphylococcus aureus meningitis. Quart J Med 53:289, 1984.
3. Gold R: Bacterial meningitis - 1982. Am J Med 75(1B):98, 1983.
4. Kaplan SL: Antigen detection in cerebrospinal fluid - pros and cons. Am J Med 75(1B):109, 1983.
5. Lavetter A, Leedom JM, Mathies AW Jr, Ivler D, Wehrle PF: Meningitis due to listeria monocytogenes. A review of 25 cases. N Engl J Med 285:598, 1971.
6. Public Health Advisory Committee on Immunization Practices - Meningococcal polysaccharide vaccines. Ann Intern Med 89:949, 1978.
7. Tauber MG, Sande MA: Principles in the treatment of bacterial meningitis. Am J Med 76:224, 1984.

A MIDDLE-AGED WOMAN WITH AN ABNORMAL GAIT

CASE 42: A 43-year-old woman was seen because of a gait disorder and paresthesias. Two years earlier she was noted to be anemic and the diagnosis of thallassemia was made on the basis of a hemoglobin electrophoresis. One year earlier she developed paresthesias and noted a change in her mood. Neurologic examination at that time was normal. She had no neck pain, injury, or Lhermitte symptom. At this time her mental status examination was notable for extreme tearfulness which, according to her family, was a definite change from her usual state. There was spasticity of both legs with normal strength. Reflexes were increased at the knees and absent at the ankles. Plantar responses were extensor. Vibration and small joint position sensation was absent in the legs and moderately reduced in the arms. Rapid alternating movements and finger-to-nose testing were normal. Gait was unstable and she required assistance to walk. The Romberg test was positive. Laboratory studies included a hematocrit of 35% with a mean corpuscular volume (MCV) of 138. CSF examination, spinal X-rays, and complete myelogram were normal. A blood smear is shown below:

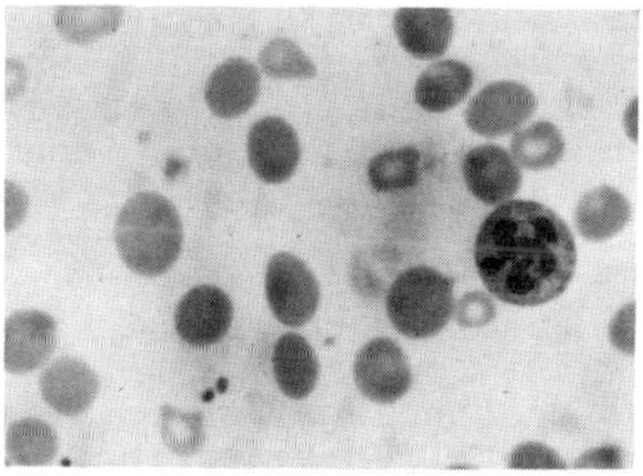

QUESTIONS:

1. What is the significance of the hematologic abnormality in this patient?
2. How can the correct diagnosis be established?
3. What are the different underlying causes of this patient's disease?
4. What are the neurologic manifestations of this disease? Cutaneous? Gastrointestinal?
5. How should this patient be treated? What is her prognosis?

ANSWERS:

1. The blood smear shows macrocytosis, anisocytosis, and a hypersegmented polymorphonuclear leukocyte. These findings are commonly seen in patients with megaloblastic anemia, usually due to a deficiency of vitamin B_{12} or folic acid.

2. A serum B_{12} level would likely be low in this patient; this test occasionally gives falsely normal values and thus in suspect cases with "normal" B_{12} levels (by RIA), a microbiological assay for vitamin B_{12} and/or Schilling test should be performed. Subacute combined degeneration, a neurologic syndrome due to a deficiency of vitamin B_{12}, was the diagnosis in this patient.

3. Most patients with B_{12} deficiency have pernicious anemia, i.e., deficient intrinsic factor production by the stomach. Intrinsic factor is necessary for vitamin B_{12} transport across the gut wall. Less commonly, B_{12} deficiency results from disease of the ileum, the site of B_{12} absorption. Thus, patients with Crohn's disease, sprue and other malabsorption syndromes, and bacterial overgrowth postgastrectomy syndromes may develop B_{12} deficiency. A Schilling test can separate those patients with intrinsic factor deficiency from those who have impaired absorption of vitamin B_{12} due to intestinal disease.

4. a) Neurologic - The myelopathy of subacute combined degeneration involves the posterior and lateral columns; clinically, patients first complain of paresthesias in the legs, associated with loss of position and vibration sensation. Pyramidal symptoms (weakness and spasticity of the legs) are also present in most patients. Visual complaints and optic atrophy may occur and are usually symmetric. Mental status changes, including irritability, somnolence, confusion, and paranoia, may also be seen. Most patients have a mild peripheral neuropathy with absent ankle jerks. The Romberg sign is usually positive in this disease. b) Cutaneous - Patients typically have a yellow pallor to the skin and a sore tongue (glossitis) with a loss of normal tongue papillations. c) Gastrointestinal - Anorexia, abdominal pain, and diarrhea may occur. Patients with pernicious anemia have, in addition, gastric achlorhydria and have a high incidence of gastric cancer.

5. Intramuscular <u>injections</u> of vitamin B_{12} will prevent the progression of neurological symptoms and, in early cases of subacute combined degeneration, will cause a complete reversal of the signs and symptoms.

PEARLS:

1. Pernicious anemia is usually seen in middle-aged, light-skinned persons of Northern European (particularly Scandinavian) descent; 25% of patients with pernicious anemia have a positive family history for that disease. Look for other manifestations of autoimmune diseases, such as vitiligo, hypothyroidism, or adrenal insufficiency.

2. A <u>myelopathy</u> similar to subacute combined degeneration may occur in patients who are not vitamin B_{12} deficient. In those patients, pyramidal signs <u>precede</u> posterior column signs, unlike the situation with B_{12} deficiency.

3. <u>Cervical spondylosis</u> is the most common cause of extensor plantar responses and loss of posterior column function in the elderly, but does not usually cause absent ankle jerks.

4. The <u>paresthesias</u> of B_{12} deficiency may be painful or complex (sensation of bugs crawling or water dripping on legs).

5. The <u>neuropathology</u> of subacute combined degeneration consists of patchy disruption of myelin.

6. Neurological symptoms develop in up to 95% of untreated patients with B_{12} deficiency.

PITFALLS:

1. Other diseases which can mimic the myelopathy of B_{12} deficiency include multiple sclerosis, cervical spondylosis, spinal cord tumors, and neurosyphilis (tabes dorsalis).

2. The hematologic but <u>not</u> neurologic symptoms of B_{12} deficiency will improve following dietary supplemenation with multivitamins containing folate. The neurologic manifestations of B_{12} deficiency may also occur in patients with a normal hematocrit.

3. Patients with a <u>definite sensory level</u> are unlikely to have a metabolic or degenerative disease such as B_{12} deficiency.

4. Question the diagnosis of subacute combined degeneration in patients with <u>asymmetrical</u> neurologic findings.

5. In patients with pernicious anemia, frequent tests for occult stool blood are important to detect early the presence of gastric carcinoma.

REFERENCES

1. Agamanolis DP, et al: Neuropathology of experimental vitamin B_{12} deficiency in monkeys. Neurology 26:905, 1976.
2. Babior BM, Bunn HF: Megaloblastic anemias. In <u>Harrison's Principles of Internal Medicine</u>, Petersdorf, et al (Eds), 10th edition. New York, McGraw-Hill, pp. 1853-1860, 1983.
3. Fairbanks VF, Elveback LR: Tests for pernicious anemia: Serum vitamin B_{12} assay. Mayo Clin Proc 58:135-137, 1983.
4. Silberstein EB: The Schilling test. JAMA 208:3235, 1969.
5. Victor M, Lear AA: Subacute combined degeneration of the spinal cord. Am J Med 20:896, 1956.

PROGRESSIVE WEAKNESS AND UNREACTIVE PUPILS IN A WAITER

CASE 43: A 47-year-old Yugoslavian-born waiter was admitted with ptosis and dysphagia. Eight days earlier he ate a "bad steak" in the evening. While at work the following day he drank two cups of soup from a large stock continuously warmed for customers. That evening nausea, vomiting, and abdominal bloating began. Two days later he noted diplopia and examination in a local emergency room showed pupillary paralysis and bilateral sixth nerve palsies. Tetracycline was prescribed but could not be ingested because he rapidly developed a dry, painful throat. Three days prior to admission his eyelids drooped and the dysphagia worsened. A neurological consultant described bilateral ptosis in addition to the above findings. Tensilon and Schick tests were negative. Lumbar puncture revealed normal opening pressure, acellular CSF, and normal glucose and protein contents. He was transferred to the hospital.

On admission, he appeared acutely ill. Blood pressure 85/60, pulse 80, temperature 99.8 pr. The mouth was dry and the oropharynx red. The abdomen was distended and hypertympanitic. Speech was hoarse. The pupils were 8 mm in diameter without direct or consensual light responses. There was bilateral ptosis and a symmetric decrease in both vertical and horizontal gaze. Facial sensation was normal. Upper facial movements were 7/10; lower were 10/10. Movements of the tongue and palate were normal. Motor examination revealed moderate symmetrical weakness of the arms against resistance; tendon reflexes were within normal limits and plantar responses were flexor. Sensory and cerebellar examinations were unremarkable.

QUESTIONS:

1. Why is this patient unlikely to have myasthenia gravis? Guillain-Barre syndrome?

2. What diagnosis is most likely in this patient and what treatment should be given?

ANSWERS:

1. Dilated, unreactive pupils are not seen in myasthenia gravis; areflexia is a hallmark of Guillain-Barré syndrome and was not present in this patient.

2. The rapidly progressive syndrome of bulbar followed by generalized weakness without sensory loss, the dilated, unreactive pupils, and the constipation are typical of botulism poisoning. Although most cases of botulism today are due to improperly home canned food, botulism can occur after consumption of poorly stored, partially cooked foods. In this patient, diagnosis was confirmed by the passive transmission of disease by serum and feces to mice and by the protection of those mice by specific antitoxin. Electromyogram (EMG) demonstrated a pattern of "jitter" and facilitation of amplitude with repeated stimulation; these findings are typical of botulism. Treatment consists of vigorous respiratory and other supportive care and administration of botulism antitoxin.

QUESTIONS:

1. Three important, although uncommon, neurologic disorders - diphtheria, botulism, and tetanus - are due to the actions of bacterial toxins. What clinical features suggest diptheria infection? Botulism? Tetanus?

2. What is the site of action of each of these toxins which account for their respective clinical syndromes?

ANSWERS:

1. a) Diphtheria - pharyngeal inflammation with palatal paralysis followed by other cranial nerve motor and sensory signs (2-3 weeks); a late sensorimotor neuropathy (5-8 weeks) may follow. Alternatively, the site of infection can be a wound or other skin lesion and in those cases the neurologic symptoms may first appear locally. b) Botulism - nausea, vomiting, and constipation followed by blurred vision and diplopia with dilated, unreactive pupils; other cranial nerve findings and progressive motor weakness follow (2-4 days). c) Tetanus - trismus, followed by spasms and rigidity of bulbar musculature and generalized muscular contractions. Local forms of tetanus can also occur.

2. a) Diphtheria - demyelinating neuropathy; this explains the motor *and* sensory findings. b) Botulism - effects of toxin at neuromuscular junction, presynaptic portion, inhibiting acetylcholine release (site of pathology similar to Eaton-Lambert syndrome); this explains the motor *without* sensory signs. c) Tetanus - interference with reflex arcs by suppressing inhibitory neurons (analogous to strychnine poisoning); this explains the spasms.

PEARLS:

1. The *cranial nerves* are usually affected first in botulism, diphtheria, and tetanus.

2. Eye findings in diphtheria include loss of accommodation with reactive pupils ("ciliary paralysis"); this is the reverse of the Argyll Robertson pupil of neurosyphilis.

3. Paresthesias and rapidly progressive generalized weakness with nausea and vomiting may occur with shellfish poisoning ("red tide").

4. Progressive, ascending motor paralysis may be due to the effects of a neurotoxin elaborated by tics (tic paralysis).

PITFALLS:

1. The sensorimotor paralysis of diphtheria and the motor paralysis of botulism may resemble Guillain-Barré syndrome (GBS) and, in particular, the Fisher variant of GBS.

REFERENCES

1. Cherrington M: Botulism: 10 year experience. Arch Neurol 30:432, 1974.
2. Cherrington M, Ryan DW: Botulism and guanidine. N Engl J Med 278:931, 1968.
3. Fisher CM, Adams RD: Diphtheric polyneuritis: A pathologic study. J Neuropath Exp Neurol 15:243, 1976.
4. Metzger JF, Lewis GE Jr: Human-derived immunoglobulins for the treatment of botulism. Rev Infect Dis 1:689, 1979.
5. Rapoport S, Watkins PB: Descending paralysis resulting from occult wound botulism. Ann Neurol 16:359, 1984.
6. Tacket CO, Shandera WX, Mann JM, Hargrett NJ, Blake PA: Equine antitoxin use and other factors that predict outcome in type A food-borne botulism. Am J Med 76:794, 1984.
7. Weinstein L: Current concepts: Tetanus. N Engl J Med 289:1293, 1973.

CONFUSION AND CRANIAL NERVE ABNORMALITIES

CASE 44: A 37-year-old summer camp director was well until 6 months previously when he developed headaches and two brief episodes of diplopia which resolved spontaneously. Ophthalmologic examination was normal. Two months previously his headaches became worse and were associated with episodic vomiting. His family noted intermittent confusion and poor memory. He was thought to be suffering from depression, but a trial of antidepressants was ineffective. One week previously he was noted to be more confused and was hospitalized.

On examination, he was a thin, diaphoretic man who was markedly confused and confabulated that the examiner was his brother. He was disoriented to place and amnestic to recent events. Speech was clear and there was no dysphasia present. He could carry out one-step, but not two-step, commands. His visual acuity was normal. There was bilateral papilledema. Cranial nerve testing revealed limited lateral rectus function bilaterally and a right facial paresis of the lower motor neuron type. Strength and sensation were intact. Reflexes were hyperactive in the legs and plantar responses were extensor. Gait was markedly ataxic and he required assistance to walk. Routine hematology and chemistry values were normal. A CT scan was performed and is pictured below. Following the CT scan, a lumbar puncture revealed an opening pressure of 650 mm H_2O, 42 lymphocytes/mm^3, a protein of 375 mg%, and glucose of 30 mg%.

NEUROANATOMICAL CLUE:

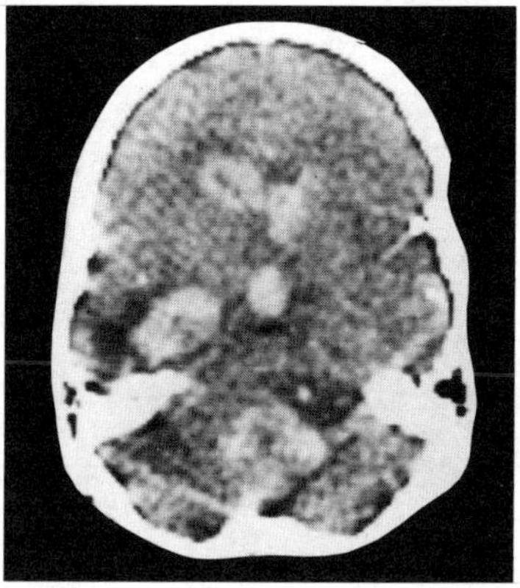

QUESTIONS

1. What is your interpretation of the CT scan findings?

2. What CNS tumors commonly present with this picture? What is the most likely diagnosis?

3. What diagnostic studies would you suggest?

4. What are the major modes of presentation of this disease?

5. What groups of individuals are particularly susceptible to this tumor?

ANSWERS:

1. The CT scan shows diffuse enhancement surrounding the 3rd, 4th, and lateral ventricles. This indicates that the blood-brain barrier is diffusely disrupted along the ventricular surface.

2. The CT scan is consistant with a primary central nervous system lymphoma or with metastatic carcinoma to the meninges (meningeal carcinomatosis). Occasionally, other chronic infectious or inflammatory diseases can mimic this CT scan picture. Because of the chronic (6-month) evolution of this patient's complaints, CNS lymphoma is more likely than metastatic carcinoma.

3. A meningeal/brain biopsy is indicated to establish the diagnosis. In this patient, meningeal and parenchymal lymphoma was found.

4. Primary CNS lymphoma has two major presentations: a) meningeal/cerebral - chronic meningitis, focal signs, and cranial nerve palsies (esp. VII, III, IV, and VI); b) solitary mass lesion in the hemispheres or posterior fossa.

5. Patients with immunodeficiency states are most susceptible to primary CNS lymphomas; groups at increased risk are those with renal transplants, congenital immunodeficiency syndromes, following therapy for Hodgkin's disease, autoimmune diseases, and, recently, acquired immunodeficiency syndrome (AIDS).

PEARLS:

1. The usual presentation of systemic lymphoma which is secondarily metastatic to the CNS is that of extradural spinal cord or brain compression.

2. Clues to the presence of lymphoma in CNS are: a) picture of aseptic meningitis with markedly elevated protein; b) a homogeneous mononuclear morphology of CSF cells.

3. The pathologic extent of CNS lymphoma is more widespread than the symptoms and signs would suggest.

4. CNS lymphoma is steriod-sensitive and radiosensitive.

5. Primary CNS lymphomas represent 1% of lymphomas in the general population and 50% of lymphomas in patients following renal transplantation.

PITFALLS:

1. The CT scan of lymphoma may mimic that of multiple sclerosis.

2. The diagnosis of CNS lymphoma is particularly difficult if spontaneous remissions have occurred.

3. The morphology of CSF cells in CNS lymphoma may appear histologically normal and should not dissuade one from the correct diagnosis.

REFERENCES

1. Adams RD: Certain notable clinical attributes of the histiocytic sarcomas of the central nervous system. Acta Neuropathol (Suppl)(Berl) 6:177, 1975.
2. Henry JM, Heffner RR Jr., Dillard SH, et al: Primary malignant lymphomas of the central nervous system. Cancer 34:1293, 1974.
3. Hochberg FH, et al: Central nervous system lymphoma related to Epstein-Barr virus. N Engl J Med 309:745, 1983.
4. Karcher KH, Jentzsch K: Radiotherapy of malignant lymphomas. Acta Neuropathol (Suppl)(Berl) 6:217, 1975.
5. Lehrich JR, Hedley-White ET, Harris ML: Acquired immunodeficiency syndrome and cranial nerve abnormalities (Case records of the MGH). N Engl J Med 309:359, 1983.
6. Raz I, Siegal T, Siegal T, Polliack A: CNS involvement by non-Hodgkin's lymphoma. Response to a standard therapeutic protocol. Arch Neurol 41:1167, 1984.
7. Schaumburg HH, Plank CR, Adams RD: The reticulum cell sarcoma-microglioma group of brain tumors. A consideration of the clinical features and therapy. Brain 95:195, 1972.
8. Schneck SA, Penn I: De-novo brain tumours in renal transplant recipients. Lancet 1:983, 1971.
9. Singh A, Strobos RJ, Singh EM, et al: Steroid-induced remissions in CNS lymphoma. Neurology 32:1267, 1982.
10. Williams RS, Crowell RM, Fisher CM, Davis K, Lavyne MH, Ropper AH, Bremer AM: Clinical and radiologic remission in reticulum cell sarcoma of the brain. Arch Neurol 36:206, 1979.

TWO PATIENTS WITH ATAXIA

<u>CASE 45</u>:

A) A 17-year-old girl was admitted because of ataxia. At age 11 she noted mild imbalance during athletics at school; over the next 5 years her imbalance became progressively more noticeable and for the past year she had been unable to walk without a cane. Two years previously she developed shakiness of her hands and deterioration of her handwriting. She is one of four children; an older brother had a similar illness, was bedridden by his late teens, and died at age 22 of pneumonia. The family is of Italian origin and without other history of neurologic disease.

General examination was remarkable for pes cavus and "hammer toe" deformities.

On neurologic examination, she was alert and intelligent. Speech was dysarthric. There was ocular dysmetria. Cranial nerve function was otherwise normal. Her gait was broad-based and markedly ataxic; she was unable to walk more than several steps without support. There was severe ataxia of all limbs on finger-to-nose and heel-to-shin testing. Reflexes were absent in the lower extremities and trace in the upper extremities; plantar responses were extensor. Position and vibration sensation were absent in the lower extremities and reduced in the upper limbs. Power was normal.

B) A 51-year-old man had a 5-year history of progressive ataxia. His first symptoms were dizziness and an unstable gait. He next noted blurred vision which was improved by an eye patch. Three years previously dysarthria and difficulty chewing food developed. An accountant, he was forced to leave his job 2 years previously because of difficulty writing. There is no family history of similar symptoms.

On examination, his speech was slow and slurred. Pupils were 3 mm and reactive; there was lateral gaze nystagmus and incomplete abduction bilaterally; vertical eye movements were intact and nystagmus was present with downgaze. Facial sensation was normal. A right facial weakness (lower motor neuron type) was present. Hearing was normal. Tongue movements were limited and the patient tended to stare and blink infrequently. Power and sensation were normal and plantar responses were flexor. There was severe ataxia on finger-to-nose and heel-to-shin maneuvers. Mild cog-wheel rigidity was present in the arms. He was wheelchair confined and unable to stand without support because of ataxia.

QUESTIONS:

1. What is ocular dysmetria? What is its significance?

2. What are the characteristics of dysarthria from cerebellar disease? Upper motor neuron (corticobulbar) disease? Lower motor neuron disease?

3. In case A, what is the significance of the areflexia? What is the most likely diagnosis?

4. What areas of the nervous system are affected in case B?

5. The CT scan from case B is shown below. What is the most likely diagnosis?

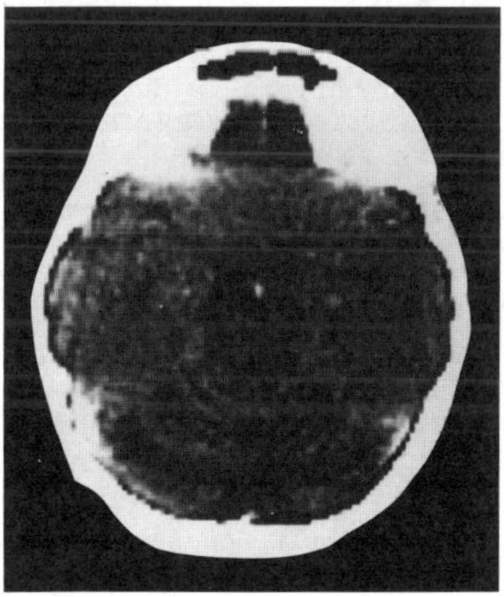

ANSWERS:

1. Ocular dysmetria is elicited by asking a patient to look laterally and then rapidly back to the midline; with ocular dysmetria, there is an overshoot of the midline followed by multiple back and forth oscillations until midline gaze is achieved. Ocular dysmetria is a symptom of cerebellar disease and is phenomenologically similar to limb dysmetria.

2. a) Cerebellar or scanning speech consists of abnormalities in rhythm (staccato), volume (poor modulation), and accentuation (emphasis placed on the wrong syllable or word). Patients with scanning speech often sound as if they are speaking English with a foreign accent. b) Spastic dysarthria from corticobulbar tract disease is usually seen in patients with pseudobulbar palsy (pathological emotions, hyperactive bulbar reflexes, bifacial weakness, dysphagia). Spastic speech is slow, "stiff," and indistinct. c) Patients with lower motor neuron disease or with muscle disease have a slurred, nasal quality to their speech, and patients with extrapyramidal disease, such as Parkinson's disease, have a low-pitched, often whispered, slurred, monotonous speech.

3. Areflexia in this patient is due to dorsal root ganglia and peripheral nerve involvement. Friedreich's ataxia is the most common cause of familial ataxia in adolescence or young adulthood. Friedreich's ataxia is a "spinocerebellar" ataxia which affects predominantly the spinal cord and not the cerebellum itself. In addition, there is a concomitant peripheral neuropathy and frequently pes cavus and hammer toe deformities. Cardiac abnormalities, including conduction disturbances, are common and may cause sudden death. Friedreich's ataxia, in some families, has been reported to be associated with an abnormality of pyruvate metabolism, specifically the enzyme lipoamide dehydrogenase.

4. Cerebellar or cerebellar connections (gait and limb ataxia), corticospinal tract (extensor plantar responses), brainstem (dizziness, facial paralysis, 6th nerve palsy, downbeat nystagmus), and extrapyramidal system (rigidity, cog-wheeling, decreased blink).

5. The CT scan shows atrophy of the pons and cerebellum. These are typical findings of olivopontocerebellar degeneration (OPCD), a degenerative disease affecting the inferior olives, pontine nuclei, and cerebellum. In some cases of OPCD, parkinsonian-like symptoms are prominent. This disease can be either familial or, as in this case, sporadic.

PEARLS

1. Multiple sclerosis is an important cause of ataxia in young adults.

2. The onset of progressive ataxia in late life may be due to nutritional deficiency states (including chronic alcoholism) or be due to an occult neoplasm.

3. An autosomal dominant disease similar to OPCD but with less severe limb ataxia has been described in Portuguese families from the Azores (Machado-Joseph disease or Azorean disease).

4. Hypotonia can be a sign of cerebellar disease and is ipsilateral to the lesion.

5. Excellent recovery may follow complete removal of a cerebellar hemisphere, particularly in children.

PITFALLS

1. Not all ataxia is due to disease of the cerebellum itself. Ataxia may be a sign of brainstem, spinal cord, or peripheral nerve disease. Remember that the cerebellum is histologically normal in patients with Friedreich's ataxia.

2. Think of hypothyroidism as a cause of progressive ataxia (via peripheral neuropathy).

3. Many eponyms and classifications have been used to describe and to "split" different subgroups of hereditary ataxias. At this time, these classifications have little therapeutic relevance and, within affected kindreds, individual variations and overlap syndromes may occur. Spinocerebellar degeneration is a good term to describe this group of disorders.

REFERENCES

1. Allen JH, Martin JT, McLain LW: Computed tomography and cerebellar atrophic processes. Radiology 130:379, 1979.
2. Gilman S, Bloudell J, Lechtenberg R: Disorders of the Cerebellum. Contemporary Neurology Series, Vol. 21. Philadelphia, F.A. Davis, 1981.
3. Harding AE: Friedreich's ataxia: a clinical and genetic study of 90 families with an analysis of early diagnostic criteria and intra-familial clustering of clinical features. Brain 104:589, 1981.
4. Konigsmark BW, Weiner LP: The olivopontocerebellar atrophies: A review. Medicine (Baltimore) 49:227, 1970.
5. Lechtenberg R, Gilman S: Speech disorders in cerebellar disease. Ann Neurol 3:285, 1978.
6. Rodriguez-Budelli M, Kark P: Kinetic evidence for a structural abnormality of lipoamide-dehydrogenase in two patients with Friedreich ataxia. Neurology 28:1283, 1978.
7. Romanul FCA, Fowler HL, Radvan J, Feldman RG, Reingold M: Azorean disease of the nervous system. N Engl J Med 296:1505, 1977.

HEADACHE AND PAPILLEDEMA IN A YOUNG MAN

CASE 46: A 32-year-old recently married lawyer was well until 4 months previously when he developed intermittent headaches described as "not throbbing, but deep in my head." Typically, headaches were present when he first awakened in the morning and recurred periodically throughout the day. He also reported having difficulty "concentrating" at work, but attributed that to the headaches and to the pressure of his job. One month previously he visited a neurologist, at which time examination was within normal limits and a lumbar puncture revealed: opening pressure 240 mm H_2O, acellular, clear fluid, protein 84 mg%, glucose 70 mg%. No cause for his symptoms could be determined and he now comes for a second opinion at the urging of his wife who noted subtle personality changes.

Examination reveals a tall, muscular, healthy-appearing young man who is bright, alert, and cooperative. Fundoscopic examination reveals blurring of disc margins bilaterally consistent with papilledema. The remainder of the neurological examination is normal.

QUESTIONS:

1. Why is the patient unlikely to have pseudotumor cerebri (see case 14)? What further workup, if any, would you recommend?

2. A CT scan was performed and is shown below. What is your impression of the CT scan?

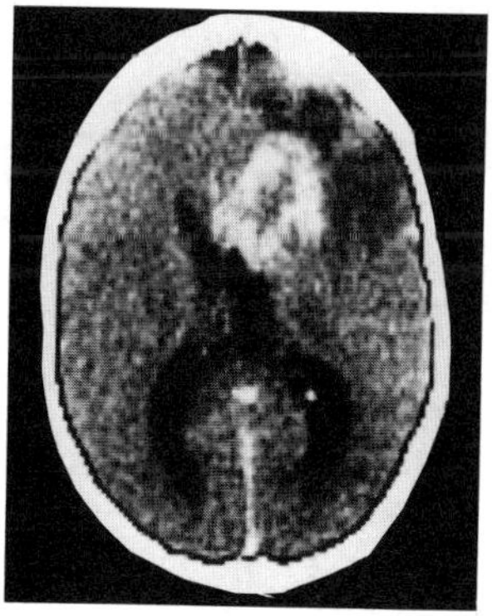

ANSWERS:

1. Patients with pseudotumor generally have decreased, _not_ increased CSF protein values; pseudotumor cerebri is a diagnosis of exclusion in patients who are not found to have focal CNS disease to account for their symptoms of headache and raised intracranial pressure. Because of the recent onset of papilledema in this patient and the elevated CSF protein, a CT scan was indicated.

2. The contrast-enhanced CT scan demonstrates a _right frontal mass_; this picture is characteristic of _malignant glioma_.

QUESTIONS:

1. What are the common presenting symptoms of brain tumor in adults?

2. What treatment is indicated?

3. What is the prognosis for this patient?

4. What are possible causes of this disease?

ANSWERS:

1. The three most common presentations of brain tumor in adults are: a) headache; b) focal seizures or other neurologic sign; c) subtle personality or intellectual changes.

2. Symptomatic therapy to reduce intracranial pressure and relieve headache is indicated. Corticosteroids, typically dexamethasone 10 mg IV bolus followed by 4 mg po q6h, is the drug of choice. If signs of raised intracranial pressure persist, dehydrating agents (glycerol and mannitol) may be necessary. Surgical therapy generally consists of a subtotal resection followed by radiotherapy. In some clinical trials, chemotherapy is added, usually including BCNU. Although chemotherapy appears to prolong survival, its value in appreciably improving the overall outlook for patients has not been established.

3. The prognosis for maligant glioma is very poor; less than 20% of patients survive 12 months following diagnosis and cure is not a reasonable goal of therapy at this time.

4. Carcinogens, in particular methylcholanthrene and nitrosoureas (rubber manufacturing), are implicated as risk factors for cerebral gliomas. Viruses are also suspected of playing a role in glioma development and multifocal gliomas are known to occur in association with progressive multifocal leukoencephalopathy (PML).

PEARLS

1. Tumors in the frontal lobes, nondominant parietal lobe, and in the thalamus may grow to a large extent before producing symptoms.

2. The onset of a focal seizure disorder in adulthood should suggest the possibility of brain tumor.

3. The duration between onset of symptoms and diagnosis is typically 3-6 months in patients with malignant glioma. In patients with low-grade astrocytoma, the duration may be several years.

4. Most brain tumors in adults are <u>supratentorial</u>; most tumors in children are <u>infratentorial</u>.

5. Less malignant gliomas (<u>astrocytomas</u>) are associated with a longer life expectancy but not with cure. Such tumors tend to become histologically and biologically more malignant with time.

PITFALLS

1. Gliomas tend to be multifocal and to infiltrate diffusely. This has been the major impediment to complete resection and surgical cure.

2. Every patient with a recent personality change needs a thorough neurologic investigation. Family members are often the best historians in such situations.

3. In patients with brain tumor, the attitudes of physicians and families range from the very aggressive to nihilistic. <u>In almost all cases</u>, surgical biopsy is indicated to establish the diagnosis and to rule out other more treatable conditions, such as infection and meningioma.

4. Patients and families of patients with brain tumor need symptomatic medical and emotional support.

5. Some astrocytomas may be missed with initial CT scan (with contrast) and only later picked up by serial scans, or by magnetic resonance imaging.

REFERENCES

1. Farwell J, Flannery JT: Cancer in relatives of children with central nervous system neoplasms. N Engl J Med 311:749, 1984.
2. Frankel SA, German WJ: Glioblastoma multiforme: A review of 219 cases with regard to natural history, pathology, diagnostic method and history. J Neurosurg 15:489, 1958.
3. Grufin von Einsiedel H: Nuclear magnetic resonance imaging of brain tumours unrevealed by CT. Europ J Radiol 2:226, 1982.
4. Hochberg SH, Pruitt A: Assumptions in the radiotherapy of glioblastoma. Neurology 30:907, 1980.
5. Shapiro, WR: Treatment of neuroectodermal brain tumors. Ann Neurol 12:231, 1982.
6. Walker AE, Robins M, Weinfeld FD: Epidemiology of brain tumors: the national survey of intracranial neoplasms. Neurology 35:219, 1985.
7. Walker MD, Greene SB, Byar DP, et al: Randomized comparisons of radiotherapy and nitrosoureas for the treatment of malignant glioma after surgery. N Engl J Med 303:1323, 1980.
8. Wilson CB: Brain tumors. N Engl J Med 300:1469, 1979.
9. Wulff JD, et al: False-negative CT's in astrocytomas: The value of repeat scanning. Neurology (NY) 32:766, 1982.

LOW BACK PAIN IN A YOUNG MAN

CASE 47: A 21-year-old man developed sudden low back pain "shooting" into the left leg when he jumped off a truck 3 weeks previously. The pain was described as excruciating, midline, and exacerbated by walking or by sudden movements of his back; the pain radiated down his posterior thigh and into his foot. He also complained of intermittent paresthesias of his left great toe. Coughing or sneezing increased the pain. There were no changes in bowel or bladder function. Initial treatment by his internist consisted of complete bedrest for 2 weeks; although the pain decreased with bedrest, it returned with ambulation.

Observation and palpation of the lower back was unrevealing. With the patient lying flat, there was severe back and left leg pain on straight-leg raising when his left leg was raised 20°. On raising his right leg 45°, left leg pain also appeared. Strength and sensation in his left leg were normal. There was a decreased ankle jerk on the left. Rectal tone, anal wink, and bulbocavernous reflex were intact.

On the following 2 pages, a schematic view of the spinal roots and this patient's myelogram are shown.

QUESTIONS:

1. What is the significance of the crossed straight-leg raising test? Of the decreased ankle jerk on the left?

2. What are the symptoms which occur with compression of the S1 root? L5 root? L4 root?

3. What are the pathophysiologic mechanisms responsible for symptoms in this patient?

4. What is appropriate management for this patient?

5. What are the symptoms of a lesion of the cauda equina? Conus medullaris? What are the usual causes of these syndromes?

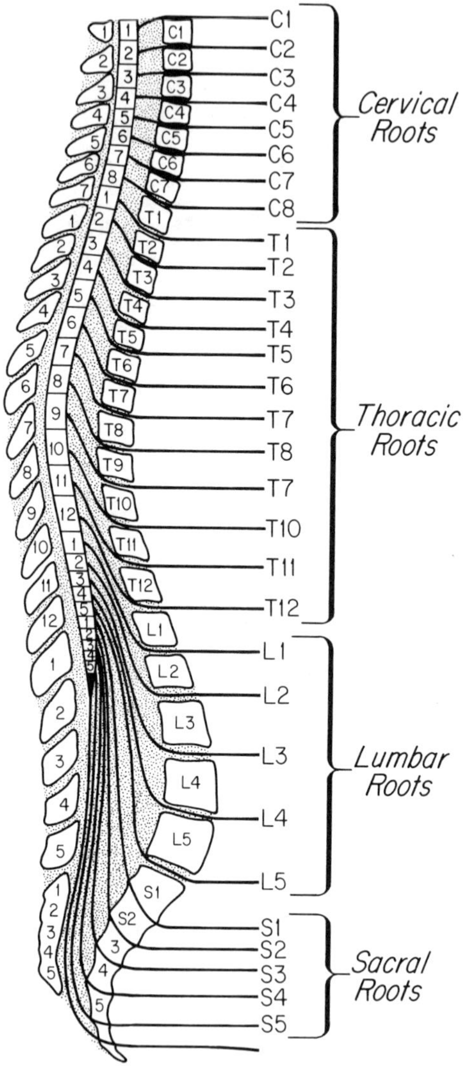
C1
C2
C3
C4
C5
C6
C7
C8
Cervical Roots
T1
T2
T3
T4
T5
T6
T7
T8
T7
T10
T11
T12
Thoracic Roots
L1
L2
L3
L4
L5
Lumbar Roots
S1
S2
S3
S4
S5
Sacral Roots

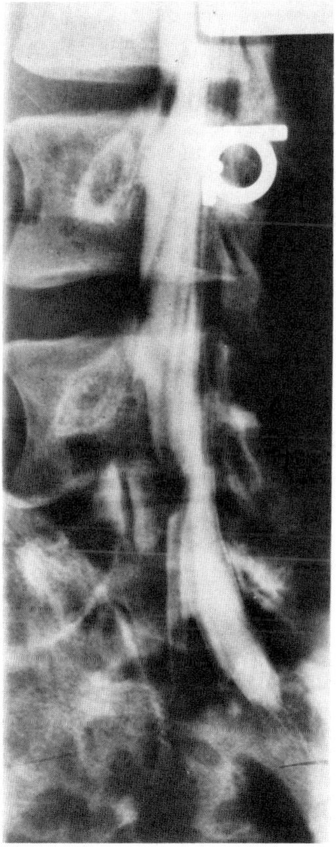

ANSWERS:

1. A positive crossed straight-leg raising test (in this patient the development of pain down the left leg with raising of the right leg) is highly suggestive of a compressive root lesion. A decreased ankle jerk suggests involvement of the S1 root.

2. S1 root (e.g., due to L5-S1 disc) - pain radiates down the posterior leg and into the fourth and fifth toes; sensory symptoms affect the lateral calf, foot, and fourth and fifth toes; motor involvement affects the extensors of ankles (gastrocnemius); diminished ankle jerk. L5 root (L4-5 disc) - pain radiates down the posterior thigh, lateral calf, and into the great toe; sensory symptoms affect the lateral calf and great toe and motor symptoms involve the extensors of great toe; reflexes normal. L4 root (L3-4 disc) - pain and sensory symptoms in anterior thigh; motor symptoms involve the quadriceps; diminished knee jerk.

3. Roots are usually compressed by nucleus pulposus material which herniates posteriorly into the spinal canal. Alternatively, osteophytes can compress roots at their exit from the vertebral foramina. Both mechanisms may be present in some patients, and disc herniation may foster the growth of foraminal osteophytes.

4. A second 2-week course of bedrest failed to significantly reduce this patient's symptoms and a myelogram was then performed which revealed a large left-sided L5-S1 disc. Surgery was performed with excellent results.

5. Cauda equina syndromes present as low back pain and progressive, asymmetric paralysis with loss of reflexes and variable sensory loss; bowel and bladder function may also be affected. Conus medullaris syndromes generally present as back pain, early and prominent bowel and bladder dysfunction, impotence, and loss of sacral reflexes. Sensory abnormalities in sacral dermatomes may be present, but motor strength is usually normal. The cauda and conus syndromes are usually due to meningioma or metastatic tumor. The cauda equina syndrome may also be due to midline lumbar disc herniation.

PEARLS:

1. The CSF protein may be mildly elevated (50-100 mg%) in disc disease.

2. X-ray findings of vertebral sclerosis or bony erosion in patients with low back pain may indicate meningioma or other tumor. Spinal X-rays may also be helpful in the patient with low back pain by detecting decreases in the width of the disc space (suggesting herniation), anterior subluxation of one vertebral body over the other (spondylolisthesis), or developmental abnormalities of the lumbosacral spine (spina bifida).

3. Neurophysiologic studies may demonstrate objective evidence of root involvement in patients with low back pain. In particular, an EMG may show segmental denervation in anterior spinal muscles or muscles of the lower extremities and nerve conduction studies may show delayed or absent late waves (H or F waves) consistent with interruption of the sensory arc.

4. A positive Babinski sign in a patient with low back pain suggests involvement of the spinal cord above L5 (vertebral body level T12-L1).

5. A single disc protrusion, especially if situated medially, may result in compression of more than one nerve root.

6. Recent advances in CT scan imaging of the lumbar spine may permit the diagnosis of herniated disc to be made in the absence of myelography.

PITFALLS:

1. Low back pain that worsens on lying down may be due to a spinal cord tumor.

2. The pain of lumbar root disease may be referred to the hip (L5 disc) or knee (L3, L4 disc) and, if not recognized, may be result in unnecessary tests and incorrect treatment.

3. The first symptoms of a retroperitoneal mass or colon or prostate carcinoma may be low back pain.

4. On occasion, an abdominal aortic aneurysm can cause back pain that mimics a herniated lumbar disc. Always check lower extremity pulses and skin temperature.

5. Evaluation of the severity of low back pain is particularly difficult, if not impossible, in patients with depression or in those involved in disability litigation.

REFERENCES

1. Friis ML, Gulliksen GC, Rasmussen P: Distribution of pain with nerve root compression. Acta Neurosurgica 39:241, 1977.
2. Hudgkins WR: The crossed straight-leg raising sign (Fajerstagn). N Engl J Med 297:1127, 1977.
3. Keim HA, Kirkaldy-Willis W: Low back pain. CIBA Clinical Symposia 32(6), 1980.
4. Raskin ST: Computed tomographic findings in lumbar disc disease. Orthopedics 5:419, 1981.

HEADACHE AND STIFF NECK

CASE 48: A 19-year-old truck driver was seen because of fever and headache. One day earlier he felt "listless" and unenergetic and complained of diffuse muscle aches. On the morning of admission, he noted chills and developed a headache, which increased in severity throughout the day. He described the headache as constant, not throbbing, and generalized. He knew of no one else who was similarly ill. There was no recent history of trauma and no prior history of significant medical illness.

Examination revealed: blood pressure 120/80; pulse 90 and regular; temperature 101.6°F. There was bilateral conjunctival effusions. There was no rash, adenopathy, or organomegaly. There was clear meningismus evoked by neck flexion. The remainder of the neurologic examination was normal.

Lumbar puncture revealed opening pressure 160 mm H_2O, clear colorless fluid. WBC 42/mm^3, 100% lymphocytes; RBC 0/mm^3. Protein 65 mg%, glucose 65/mg%.

QUESTION:

1. What is the most likely etiology for this patient's illness?

ANSWER:

1. This patient has acute aseptic meningitis, which is usually viral in origin; enteroviruses (ECHO virus, Coxsackie virus, and polio virus) and mumps virus are responsible for the vast majority of cases of viral meningitis.

QUESTIONS:

1. What clinical features suggest that acute meningitis is viral in origin?

2. What further workup is indicated?

3. How should this patient be treated?

4. Are there indications for repeat lumbar puncture in this patient?

ANSWERS:

1. Clues to a viral etiology of acute meningitis include: a virus-like prodrome, myalgias, conjunctivitis, exanthema, pleurodynia (coxsackie B virus), a similar illness in a family member or close contact.

2. CSF and blood cultures should be performed to rule out bacterial or fungal infection; liver function tests are useful to rule out coexistent hepatitis.

3. Under most circumstances, close in-hospital observation for several days is indicated, pending results of CSF and blood cultures; in certain situations, antibiotic therapy is instituted pending results of CSF cultures.

4. If bacterial cultures are negative and if the patient's clinical condition improves, no further workup is necessary and repeat lumbar puncture is not required. Diagnosis of enteroviral infection can be confirmed by isolation of the virus from stool or CSF and demonstration of an antibody titer rise.

Virus	Season	Associated Features
Enterovirus	Sporadic, with increase in Summer and Fall	May have rash, pleurodynia. Family epidemics may occur.
Mumps	Sporadic, increase in Winter and early Spring	Parotitis, orchitis, pancreatitis. Amylase frequently elevated.
Lymphocytic choriomeningitis	Fall to Winter	Carried by common mouse. Illness may be preceded by respiratory infection.
Infectious mononucleosis (Epstein-Barr virus)	Throughout year	Lymphadenopathy, may have mild hepatitis; heterophil reaction positive.
Herpes simplex type 2 (HSV2)	Throughout year	Genital lesions; transmission by venereal contact

PITFALLS:

1. In patients with acute aseptic meningitis, the main goal of treatment is to rule out treatable bacterial or fungal infections. Antibiotic therapy is appropriate for many patients with aseptic meningitis pending CSF results.

2. <u>The CSF profile in partially treated bacterial meningitis may be identical to that found in viral meningitis</u>. Although usually normal, CSF glucose may be depressed in viral meningitis (e.g., with mumps). There may be a predominance of polys in the CSF early in the course of viral meningitis.

3. <u>Leptospirosis</u> is a spirochete infection which may produce aseptic meningitis identical to that present with viral infection; leptospirosis is generally acquired by exposure to the urine of affected animals (especially rats) and many cases in the United States are acquired by vacationers at tropical beaches.

4. <u>Arboviruses</u> (arthropod-borne viruses) can cause cases of meningitis as well as fatal encephalitis in the same epidemic.

REFERENCES

1. Chonmaitree T, Menegus MA, Powell KR: The clinical relevance of "CSF viral culture": 2-years experience with aseptic meningitis in Rochester, NY. JAMA 247:1843, 1982.
2. Meningitis: aseptic or pyogenic? (editorial). Lancet 1:435, 1984.
3. Meyer HM, Johnson RT, et al: Central nervous system syndromes of "viral" etiology. Am J Med 29:334, 1960.
4. Tenser RB: Herpes simplex and herpes zoster: nervous system involvement. Neurologic clinics 2:215, 1984.

LEG WEAKNESS AND ABNORMAL CHEST X-RAY

CASE 49: A 50-year old, married woman was admitted to the hospital because of progressive left leg weakness and numbness. Review of her history revealed that 10 years previously she was told there was a "spot" on her lung and a lymph node above her clavicle was biopsied. She remained well until 6 months previously when she developed progressive weakness of her left leg and painless weakness and numbness of her left hand. She had urinary frequency without dysuria. Examination included normal vital signs and general examination, except for a firm, left supraclavicular node. Positive findings on neurologic examination included poorly reactive left pupil, weak left hand grip and left lower extremity, brisk lower extremity reflexes with upgoing toes and a sensory level to pin and touch at T8. There was profound loss of position and vibration sense in the left hand. A chest X-ray showed hilar adenopathy.

NEUROANATOMICAL CLUE: On the opposite page, a myelogram and lymph node biopsy from this patient are shown.

QUESTIONS:

1. What is the diagnosis? How was it be established? What do the myelogram and biopsy show?

2. Name the neurologic manifestations of this disease?

3. What other diseases can produce a similar granulomatous reaction in tissues?

4. What are the usual spinal fluid findings in this disease when the meninges are affected?

5. What is the appropriate treatment?

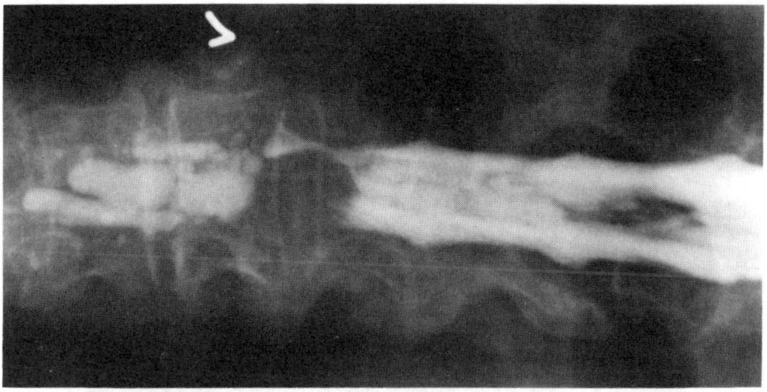

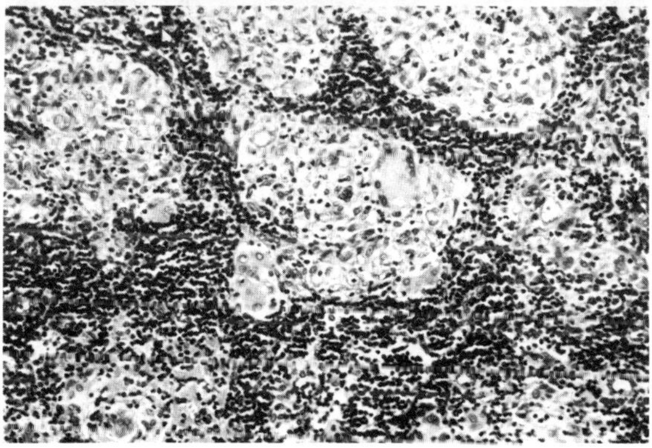

ANSWERS:

1. Spinal cord sarcoidosis. The diagnosis can be established by epidural or lymph node biopsy and by myelogram. The biopsy shows noncaseating granulomas containing giant cells; the thoracic myelogram shows an intradural, extramedullary mass displacing the spinal cord laterally. There may also be intramedullary lesions or signs of arachnoiditis in this disease.

2. Visual loss (lesions in or around optic nerve and chiasm); hydrocephalus, seizures, cranial nerve palsies (especially facial weakness); pupillary abnormalities (uveitis); corticospinal and cerebellar signs; spinal cord and meningeal involvement.

3. Protozoal infections (e.g., toxoplasmosis); fungal infections (e.g., coccidioidomycosis); spirochetal infection (e.g., *Treponema pallidum*); bacterial infection (e.g., tuberculosis, leprosy).

4. CSF lymphocytic pleocytosis (10-200 cells/mm^3); two thirds of patients have CSF proteins greater than 50 mg%. CSF gamma globulin is frequently elevated. In this case, CSF contained 20 lymphocytes/mm^3, protein was 56 mg%, and gamma globulin was 17% of total protein. Serum globulins were increased with polyclonal banding on electrophoresis.

5. Judicious use of steroids may lead to improvement or stabilization of the neurologic deficit. In this case, prednisone use did lead to improvement of hand and leg strength over the next several months.

PEARLS:

1. Remissions and long symptom-free intervals may occur in sarcoidosis even without treatment.

2. Sarcoid tubercules are frequently found in mediastinum, peripheral lymph nodes, lung, liver, and skin, and infrequently found in the central nervous system. The incidence of peripheral and/or central nervous system involvement in sarcoidosis is approximately 5%.

3. A characteristic lesion in sarcoidosis is noncaseating and contains epithelioid cells surrounded by lymphocytes and giant cells.

4. Polyuria, polydypsia, impotence, amenorrhea, somnolence, and obesity may occur due to involvement of the pituitary gland and hypothalamus.

5. Most patients with neurosarcoidosis have pre-existing systemic sarcoidosis and develop signs and symptoms of neurologic involvement during the course of their illness. This was true in this case.

PITFALLS:

1. CSF gamma globulin is frequently elevated in CNS sarcoid but, in contrast to multiple sclerosis, the serum gamma globulin is increased in the former, and normal in the latter.

2. Sarcoidosis bears a close resemblance clinically and pathologically to tuberculosis.

3. Therapy for sarcoidosis should be continued for at least 6 months and tapered "to tolerance."

4. Patients with sarcoid myelopathy may have normal myelograms; presumably small intramedullary parenchymal granulomas are present in these cases.

REFERENCES

1. Caroscio J, Yahr M: Progressive myelopathy due to sarcoid. Clin Neurol Neurosurg 82:217, 1980.
2. Day A, Sypert G: Spinal cord sarcoidosis. Ann Neurol 1:79, 1977.
3. Delaney P: Neurologic manifestations in sarcoidosis. Ann Intern Med 87:336, 1977.
4. Silverstein A, et al: Neurologic sarcoidosis. Arch Neurol 12:1, 1965.

NECK AND ARM PAIN AND LEG WEAKNESS

CASE 50: A 52-year-old man presented with complaints of neckache, right arm pain, and leg weakness. His symptoms began approximately 2 years earlier with intermittent neck aches, and then gradually progressed. There were no associated visual symptoms or bladder or bowel complaints, except for occasional nocturia. There was no incontinence. One month prior to admission he noted some weakness of his right arm. Past medical history and review of systems were otherwise unremarkable.

Examination demonstrated normal vital signs and general medical exam. There was no limitation of neck movement. On neurologic examination, mentation and cranial nerves were normal; there was no nystagmus. Motor examination revealed mild weakness of right biceps and brachioradialis and of both iliopsoas muscles (4/5). He had a diminished right biceps and brachioradialis reflex (1/4), increased right triceps (3/4), brisk knee jerks (3/4), and upgoing toes bilaterally. Sensation was normal, except for decreased position sense in both feet. Coordination was normal, and gait was somewhat spastic.

NEUROANATOMICAL CLUE: See cervical myelogram on opposite page.

QUESTIONS:

1. What is the most likely diagnosis? How can it be established?

2. What other diagnoses should be considered?

3. What is the preferred treatment for this condition?

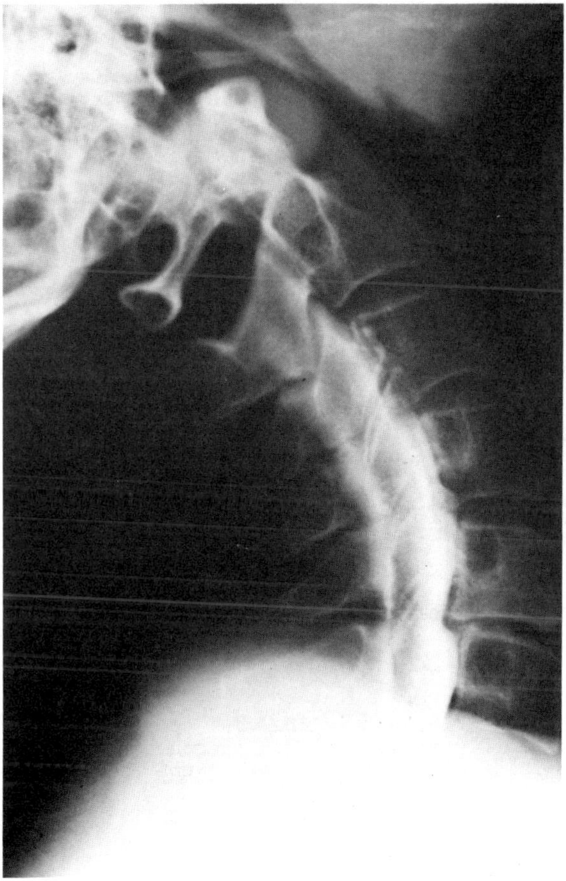

ANSWERS:

1. Cervical spondylosis and/or disc herniation at C5-6 with associated myelopathy. The diagnosis is established by cervical myelography, which in this case demonstrated a herniated cervical disc and spur between C5 and C6 compressing the cord from the front. The cord is usually compressed between osteophytes or by a disc anteriorly and by the ligamentum flavum posteriorly; cervical roots are usually compressed by bony overgrowth in the intervertebral foramina.

2. a) Multiple sclerosis - Lesions are separated in time and space. Myelogram is normal.

   b) Spinal cord tumor - May be visualized by myelography, plain films, or CT scan. CSF protein is often elevated; early bladder and bowel symptoms are common.

   c) Subacute combined degeneration due to B_{12}-deficiency - Peripheral neuropathy, macrocytic anemia, and low serum B_{12} level are expected.

   d) Syringomyelia - A "dissociated" sensory loss is expected.

3. Anterior cervical discectomy and decompression of the cord. Posterior decompression laminectomy is performed in some cases. This patient had an anterior operation and made a full recovery.

PEARLS:

1. Cervical spondylosis is the most common cause of spinal cord compression seen in general hospitals. There is often a delay in making the diagnosis.

2. Neck pain, arm pain, and leg weakness -- Think of cervical spondylosis.

3. Lower extremity spasticity is more evident than weakness in patients with cervical spondylosis and myelopathy; this is particularly true in early stages of the disease. Muscle wasting in the upper limbs is often present.

4. Bladder and bowel abnormalities occur late in cervical spondylitic myelopathy -- but early with spinal cord neoplasms or demyelinating disease.

5. Diminished biceps (C5,C6) and brachioradialis (C5,C6) reflexes and increased triceps reflexes (C7) are often clues to cervical spondylosis and myelopathy at the C5-6 interspace, causing segmental nerve root compression (C6) and pyramidal tract signs below that level ("inverted radial reflex").

PITFALLS:

1. Trauma to the cord from sudden extension of the head (fall, myelography, chiropractic manipulation) can cause sudden worsening in a case of chronic spondylosis and myelopathy.

2. Cervical spondylosis and myelopathy may mimic chronic progressive multiple sclerosis involving the spinal cord. Beware of accepting the latter diagnosis unless a cervical myelogram has been performed at some point and supportive evidence of MS exists (e.g., elevated CSF gamma globulin and/or oligoclonal bands, abnormal visual evoked response).

3. Cervical spondylosis, because it is so common, may co-exist with symptoms of other disorders (carpal tunnel syndrome, diabetic neuropathy, angina pectoris).

REFERENCES

1. Adams R, Victor M: Diseases of the spinal cord. In Principles of Neurology, New York, McGraw-Hill, pp. 634-637, 1981.
2. Brain WR, et al: The neurological manifestations of cervical spondylosis. Brain 75:187, 1952.
3. Gregorius FK, Estrain T, Crandall PH: Cervical spondylitic radiculopathy and myelopathy. A long-term followup study. Arch Neurol 33:618, 1976.
4. Lunsford LD, Bissonnette JD, Zorub DS: Anterior surgery for cervical disc disease. Part 2. Treatment of cervical spondylitic myelopathy in 32 cases. J Neurosurg 53:12, 1980.

VISUAL LOSS AND AMENORRHEA

CASE 51: A 28-year-old woman, mother of five, and wife of a farmer, was referred because of progressive visual loss of 6 months' duration. Early symptoms consisted of haziness in the right eye which over the next several weeks progressed to the point where she was unable to read or watch TV with that eye. Hazy vision had recently developed in the left eye as well. She denied double vision, weakness, sensory symptoms, or pain of any kind. There was no family history of a similar illness. Her general health was otherwise excellent, except for amenorrhea of 4 years' duration for which she had not sought medical attention and which she felt was due to having had "so many children at such a young age."

Neurologic examination revealed pallor of the right optic disc. The remainder of the cranial nerve, motor, sensory, and cerebellar examination was normal.

NEUROANATOMICAL CLUE: Visual field exam and CAT scan are shown on the opposite page.

QUESTIONS:

1. What is the significance of this patient's visual field abnormality? What area of the nervous system is implicated by this finding?
2. What is the differential diagnosis?
3. What is your interpretation of the CAT scan?
4. What additional workup is indicated?
5. What treatment is appropriate?
6. How do patients with pituitary tumors usually present?

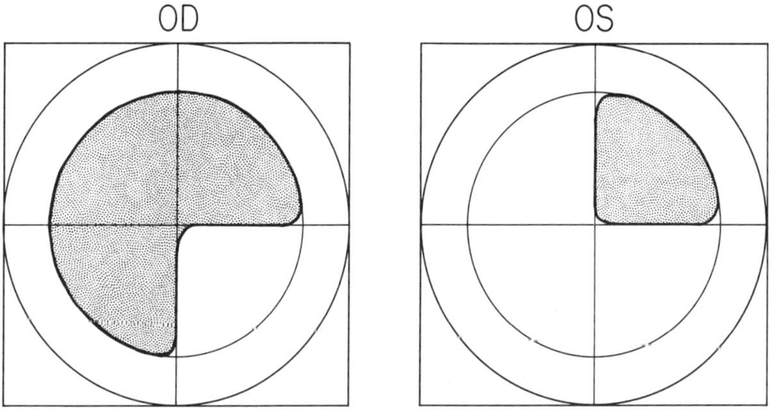
OD
OS

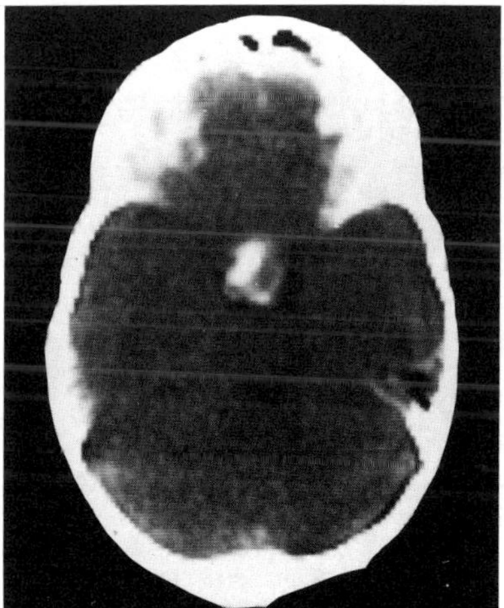

ANSWERS:

1. In the right eye there is a temporal and superior medial field cut; in the left eye there is a superior temporal field cut. Bilateral temporal visual field abnormalities suggest a lesion in the region of the optic chiasm.

2. Pituitary adenoma, aneurysm of the internal carotid artery, craniopharyngioma.

3. The CT scan shows an enhancing mass lesion in the pituitary region.

4. Arteriogram is indicated to rule out cerebral aneurysm; skull X-rays and polytomography are indicated to define the size and the presence, if any, of asymmetry and erosion of the sella turcica. In addition, a neuroendocrine evaluation and, in particular, a plasma prolactin level is indicated. These studies indicated the presence of a prolactin-producing pituitary adenoma in this patient.

5. Treatment consists of surgical removal of the pituitary adenoma, usually via a transsphenoidal approach. Some centers advocate the use of proton beam radiation in place of surgery. If the prolactin level remains elevated following surgery, or if symptoms of amenorrhea and galactorrhea persist, bromocriptine may be used to reduce prolactin levels and tumor size. The long-term prognosis is excellent.

6. Patients with pituitary tumors usually present with some combination of: a) headache; b) endocrine disturbance; c) visual disturbance.

PEARLS:

1. Visual disturbance in patients with pituitary adenoma usually involves the superior portion of the visual field before the inferior portion because the tumor compresses the optic chiasm from below.

2. Polytomography may show local bulging and erosion of the sella turcica when plain skull films and even CT scans are normal in patients with pituitary adenoma.

3. <u>Typical Endocrine Syndromes Produced by Pituitary Adenoma</u>

Syndrome	Histologic Type	Hormone Produced	Comments
Amenorrhea-galactorrhea	Chromophobe	Prolactin	In men, prolactinomas may produce impotence
Acromegaly	Chromophobe	Growth hormone	Elevated growth hormone production prior to puberty results in gigantism
Cushing's syndrome	Basophil	Adrenocorticotrophic hormone (ACTH)	Most cases of Cushing's syndrome are pituitary, not adrenal in origin

4. Significant recovery of vision follows the removal of pituitary adenomas in most patients.

PITFALLS:

1. <u>Arteriogram</u> should be performed on all patients with suspected pituitary adenoma prior to surgery in order to rule out an aneurysm of the circle of Willis.

2. Pituitary tumors (<u>microadenomas</u>) may produce endocrine symptoms without enlarging the sella turcica.

3. Depending upon the relative position of the pituitary tumor in relation to the optic chiasm, monocular blindness, bitemporal hemianopsia, or hemianopsia may result.

REFERENCES

1. Antunes JL, et al: Prolactin-secreting pituitary tumors. Ann Neurol 2:148, 1977.
2. Diayer B, et al: Diagnostic approaches to pituitary adenomas. Neurology 29:161, 1979.
3. Faria NA Jr, Tindall GT: Transsphenoidal microsurgery for prolactin-secreting pituitary adenomas: Results in 100 women with the amenorrhea-galactorrhea syndrome. J Neurosurg 56:36, 1982.
4. Koppelman MCS, et al: Hyperprolactinemia, amenorrhea, and galactorrhea: A retrospective assessment of 25 cases. Ann Intern Med 100:115, 1984.
5. McGregor AM, et al: Reduction in size of a pituitary tumor by bromocriptine therapy. N Engl J Med 300:291, 1979.
6. Nakane T, Kuwayama H, Watanabe M, Kageyana N: Transsphenoidal approach to pituitary adenomas with suprasella extension. Surg Neurol 16:225, 1981.

ALTERED BEHAVIOR AND DYSPHASIA IN AN ELDERLY WOMAN

CASE 52: A 74-year-old woman, the mother of a physician, was referred because of altered behavior and a speech disorder. She had always been a bright, witty, and verbal person, outgoing and well recognized in the community for her numerous philanthropic activities. Approximately 12 months earlier her family noted changes in her behavior, which were at first subtle and consisted of suspiciousness that her money was being mismanaged by her lawyers and by family members. Several months later she began to accuse her sons of stealing her money and of planning to send her to the Salvation Army Home to live. She began, in addition, to complain that strange men were hiding in her room, watching her dress, and stealing her underwear. At that time, changes in speech became noticeable. A slowness in talking due to word finding difficulties became progressively more disabling and over a period of months led to difficulty in comprehension as well.

A local physician, who had known the family for 20 years, told the family that the problem was "old age" and that there were nothing that could be done. The family requested a second opinion. Her past medical history was unremarkable, except for mild hypertension of 10 years' duration, treated with diuretics. There is no personal or family history of psychiatric disease nor of toxin exposure.

Examination revealed a pleasant, attentive woman, who was obviously dysphasic, with severe word finding difficulties and multiple paraphasic errors in conversation. There were deficits in comprehension of both spoken and written language; she was able to carry out one- but not two-step commands. Given a pen, she was at first unable to remove the cover and, with assistance, she wrote her name slowly and with multiple spelling errors. There was mild Geggenhalten elicited by passive arm movements and a positive snout response. Cranial nerve, motor, sensory, and reflex examinations were otherwise normal. Gait was stable and, under observation, she was able to walk up and down two flights of stairs without difficulty. Routine blood tests and electroencephalogram were normal. A CT scan was interpreted as showing ventricular dilatation and cortical atrophy.

QUESTION:

1. What is the likely diagnosis? What treatment, if any, would you recommend?

ANSWER:

1. This patient has Alzheimer's disease (senile dementia of Alzheimer's type). At present, this is an untreatable condition. Medical care is supportive, both to the patient and to the family. Occupational therapy is often helpful. In some patients with Alzheimer's disease, low dosage phenothiazine medication is helpful in controlling the abnormal behavior.

QUESTIONS:

1. Why is this patient unlikely to have aphasia secondary to a stroke?

2. Name some different presenting symptoms of Alzheimer's disease.

3. What is normal pressure hydrocephalus (NPH)? How is the diagnosis established? Why is NPH unlikely in this patient?

4. Name the important, treatable causes of dementia.

5. What is Geggenhalten? What does it signify?

ANSWERS:

1. Symptoms due to cerebrovascular disease appear *rapidly* and usually have accompanying focal motor or reflex signs; the slow progressive nature of this patient's aphasia over several months makes this symptom unlikely to be due to the effects of a stroke.

2. Forgetfulness, apraxia, aphasia, hallucinations, and behavioral changes, including paranoia, can all be presenting symptoms of Alzheimer's disease.

3. The triad of *dementia, gait disorder, and urinary incontinence* suggests normal pressure hydrocephalus. The diagnosis is supported by the finding of large ventricles on CT scan and little cortical atrophy. Clinical improvement may follow lumbar puncture. Symptoms of NPH may resolve in some patients following ventricular shunt procedures. In this patient, the normal gait and absence of urinary incontinence make NPH unlikely.

4. Meningioma, subdural hematoma, drug intoxication, hypo or hyperthyroidism, Cushing's disease, normal pressure hydrocephalus, and vitamin (B and niacin) deficiency all can produce a clinical picture of dementia. Depression can produce a picture that mimics dementia ("pseudodementia").

5. *Geggenhalten*, or fluctuating resistance to passive motion of a limb, is a sign of frontal lobe disease.

PEARLS:

1. A *CT scan* should be performed in all patients with unexplained dementia to rule out subdural hematoma, tumor, hydrocephalus, and multi-infarct dementia.

2. Early Alzheimer's disease can be confused with or complicated by *depression*. When depression exists in a patient with dementia, treatment with a course of antidepressant medication should be instituted and the effect on cognitive function monitored.

3. The prevalence of severe dementia is approximately 5% in the population past the age of 65. There are thus more than 1.3 million Americans with severe dementia, the majority of whom have Alzheimer's disease.

4. A selective decrease in choline acetyltransferase, the enzyme responsible for acetylcholine synthesis, has been found in the brains of patients with Alzheimer's disease. The significance of this finding is unknown.

5. There is an increased incidence of Alzheimer's disease in patients with _Down's_ syndrome.

6. Pathologic changes in the brains of patients with Alzheimer's disease consist of: a) a widespread _loss of nerve cells_, particularly in the cerebral cortex; b) _senile plaques_ - deposits of amorphous material in the cerebral cortex; c) _neurofibrillary tangles_ - abnormal material within the nerve cell cytoplasm; d) _granulovacuolar changes_ - vacuoles which appear in the neurons of the hippocampus.

PITFALLS:

1. Patients who complain to a physician that their memory is failing are more likely to be depressed than amnestic.

2. Difficulty walking is _not_ an early symptom of Alzheimer's disease. Furthermore, although patients with Alzheimer's disease are frequently aphasic, hemiplegia or hemianopsia are unlikely to be due to Alzheimer's disease.

3. There is no evidence that any of the manifestations of senile dementia are due to the effects of reduced cerebral blood flow. Alzheimer's disease is not "cerebral atherosclerosis".

4. A normal CT scan and normal EEG do not rule out Alzheimer's disease.

REFERENCES

1. Adams RD, Victor M: Degenerative diseases of the nervous system. In Principles of Neurology, Chap. 42, New York, McGraw-Hill, 1981.
2. Davies P, Maloney AJF: Selective loss of central cholinergic neurons in Alzheimer's disease. Lancet 2:1403, 1976.
3. Fisher CN: Hydrocephalus as a cause of disturbances of gait in the elderly. Neurology 32:1958, 1982.
4. Hubbard BN, Anderson JN: Age, senile dementia, and ventricular enlargement. J Neurol Neurosurg Psychiatry 44:631, 1981.
5. Kerzner LJ: Diagnosis and treatment of Alzheimer's disease. In Advances in Int Med 29:447, Year Book Pub (Chicago), 1984.
6. Rocci RP, et al: Recognition of dementia among medical patients. Arch Intern Med 144:73, 1984.
7. Small GW, et al: Diagnosis and treatment of dementia in the aged. West J Med 135(6):469, 1981.
8. Terry R, Katzman R: Senile dementia of the Alzheimer's type. Ann Neurol 14:497, 1983.

COMMON CLINICAL PROBLEMS

CASE 1: A 55-year-old psychotherapist awoke with weakness and numbness of the left leg; examination revealed a left foot drop (paralysis of dorsiflexion at the ankle and toes) and sensory loss on the lateral surface of the left leg.

QUESTIONS:

1. What is the correct diagnosis?

2. In what way might this be considered an occupational illness?

3. What is the appropriate therapy?

ANSWERS:

1. Peroneal nerve palsy.

2. Injury to the common peroneal nerve may occur from prolonged sitting with the legs crossed as a psychiatrist might be expected to do. Pressure on the peroneal nerve as it crosses the head of the fibula may also occur with a tight plaster cast. Alcoholics and diabetics are particularly susceptible to peroneal nerve palsy.

3. Bracing of the ankle and symptomatic therapy are appropriate.

CASE 2: A 43-year-old pianist developed pain and a pins and needles sensation in her left hand. She reports that for the past 3 months she has been awakened from sleep because of the pain radiating into her first 2 fingers and thumb. Examination was within normal limits.

QUESTIONS:

1. What is the most likely diagnosis?

2. What tests might be used to confirm the diagnosis?

3. What is the treatment for this patient's condition?

ANSWERS:

1. Carpal tunnel syndrome. Partial or intermittent compression of the median nerve in the carpal tunnel occurs commonly in individuals who use their hands extensively.

2. Clinical impression can be corroborated by reproduction of symptoms by compression of the median nerve at the wrist and by nerve conduction velocity and EMG electrical tests.

3. A cock-up wrist splint and injection of steroids into the carpal tunnel may relieve symptoms, but surgical decompression at the wrist is the most definitive treatment for this condition.

CASE 3: A 35-year-old, currently unemployed librarian is seen because of chronic, persistent headache of 15 years' duration. He reports that the headache is centered 4 inches above his left eye and 2-1/2 inches beneath his scalp. The headache has been present every waking moment for the past 15 years and has been increasing in severity over the past month. He has seen multiple physicians, had numerous unrevealing tests, and received multiple medications without satisfactory diagnosis or treatment. Neurologic examination is normal.

QUESTION:

1. What is the most likely diagnosis?

ANSWER:

1. A functional and not "organic" basis for this man's headaches is most likely.

<u>CASE 4</u>: A 52-year-old man with hypertension developed isolated diplopia on lateral gaze only.

QUESTIONS:

1. What is the most likely cause?

2. What studies are necessary?

ANSWERS:

1. Vascular infarction of a nutrient vessel to the sixth nerve related to hypertension is most likely; tumors at the base of the brain, chronic meningitis, and myasthenia gravis are less likely possibilities.

2. Determination of blood glucose, sedimentation rate, and CT scan are indicated, as is careful follow-up. Resolution over a period of several months is expected with sixth nerve palsy associated with diabetes and/or hypertension.

CASE 5: A 65 year-old man has his first generalized seizure.

QUESTIONS:

1. What should the workup involve?

2. What is the most likely etiology?

ANSWERS:

1. Noninvasive examination of carotid arteries and the cardiovascular system is indicated. In addition, determination of serum electrolytes and chemistries, examination of cerebrospinal fluid, and CT scan of the brain should be performed.

2. In this age group, the most likely cause of seizure is cerebrovascular disease with secondary brain infarction.

CASE 6: An 18-year-old, single girl was having three migraine headaches each week.

QUESTIONS:

1. What questions should you ask her?

2. What is the best prophylaxis for her headaches?

ANSWERS:

1. Is she on birth control pills? Is there a relationship between her migraine attacks and menstrual periods, diet, or stress.

2. Removal of precipatating factors, regular exercise, and, if needed, propranolol (Inderal) 60-120 mg daily. Some patients benefit from salt restriction prior to menstrual periods.

CASE 7: A 52-year-old obese woman developed numbness and burning of her left thigh. Examination revealed an area of hypalgesia along the anterolateral aspect of her left leg between the hip and knee. Power and reflexes were normal.

QUESTIONS:

1. What is the diagnosis?

2. What blood study is indicated?

ANSWERS:

1. Lateral cutaneous nerve syndrome (meralgia paraesthetica) due to infarction or compression of the (L2-3 derived) cutaneous sensory nerve. Risk factors include obesity, diabetes mellitus, and pregnancy. Mechanical compression, e.g., from tight-fitting clothes, may also be responsible.

2. Blood sugar analysis is indicated.

CASE 8: A 19-year-old woman with advanced systemic lupus erythematosus manifested by lymphadenopathy, arthralgias, renal disease, and hypertension noted the sudden development of numbness of the sole of her right foot. Examination revealed subjective changes to pinprick and light touch of the fifth toe, moderate weakness of toe and ankle flexion so that she was unable to stand on the toes of the right foot, and an absent right ankle jerk.

QUESTIONS:

1. A lesion in which nerve root is suggested by the examination?

2. What is the diagnosis?

ANSWERS:

1. S1 root.

2. Mononeuritis due to nerve infarction.

CASE 9: A 65-year-old woman with long-standing arthritis developed progressive weakness and spasticity with no change in bladder or bowel habits.

QUESTIONS:

1. What is the most likely cause?

2. What tests will establish the correct diagnosis?

ANSWERS:

1. Cervical spondylosis and secondary spinal cord compression.

2. Cervical myelography is indicated. Prior to myelography, B_{12} deficiency should be excluded in all patients.

CASE 10: A 48-year-old farmer complained of "weakness in my feet" of 6 years' duration; the weakness had slowly progressed and 1 month earlier he noted for the first time numbness in his feet as well. He recalled that his father had a similar problem and that by the age of 60 his father was able to walk only by holding on to walls or to other people. Examination revealed severe muscle atrophy and moderate muscle weakness in the lower limbs below the knee ("champagne-bottle-legs"). Sensory deficit to touch/pin was present bilaterally distal to the midcalf ("stocking-glove distribution"). Ankle jerks were absent and knee jerks trace.

QUESTIONS:

1. What clinical features suggest that this is a neuropathy rather than a myopathy?

2. What is the diagnosis?

ANSWERS:

1. Stocking-glove sensory deficit and areflexia are hallmarks of neuropathies.

2. Hereditary peroneal muscular atrophy (Charcot-Marie-Tooth disease).

Case 11: A 58-year-old woman complained of paroxysms of excruciating lancinating pains in the back of her throat and radiating to her left ear. Each episode is of extremely brief duration, but recurs several times daily. She had the identical pain 3 years ago, which lasted several months and then disappeared. The current episode began 2 weeks ago.

QUESTIONS:

1. What is the most likely diagnosis?

2. What is the appropriate treatment?

ANSWERS:

1. Glossopharyngeal neuralgia; this illness is analogous to trigeminal neuralgia, but involves the ninth rather than the fifth cranial nerve.

2. Carbamazepine or diphenylhydantoin are the treatments of choice.

CASE 12: A 23-year-old teacher was seen 10 days previously because of fever and severe headache. Because of a question of viral meningitis, a lumbar puncture was performed which was normal. The fever and constitutional symptoms improved over the following days, but her headache persisted. She complains now that the headache disappears completely when she lies in bed, but that it returns with severe intensity when she attempts to stand or walk.

QUESTIONS:

1. What is the most likely cause of this woman's headache?

2. What is the treatment and what is the prognosis?

ANSWERS:

1. Lumbar puncture headache due to chronic leakage of cerebrospinal fluid through the lumbar puncture site.

2. Intravenous and oral fluids may alleviate symptoms in many patients. The prognosis for disappearance of symptoms within 2 weeks is excellent.

Index